the FIFTH DECADE

the FIFTH DECADE

Is It Just My Life
or Is It Perimenopause?

SORTING THROUGH THE EMOTIONAL UPHEAVAL
OF WOMEN IN THEIR FORTIES AND FIFTIES

DEBORAH R. WAGNER, PH.D.

NEW YORK

the FIFTH DECADE

Is It Just My Life or Is It Perimenopause?

ISBN 978-1-61448-152-2 Paperback
ISBN 978-1-61448-153-9 eBook
Library of Congress Control Number: 2012932317

Morgan James Publishing
The Entrepreneurial Publisher
5 Penn Plaza, 23rd Floor,
New York City, New York 10001
(212) 655-5470 office • (516) 908-4496 fax
www.MorganJamesPublishing.com

Cover Design by:
Rachel Lopez
www.r2cdesign.com

Interior Design by:
Bonnie Bushman
bonnie@caboodlegraphics.com

In an effort to support local communities, raise awareness and funds, Morgan James Publishing donates a percentage of all book sales for the life of each book to Habitat for Humanity Peninsula and Greater Williamsburg.

Habitat
for Humanity®
Peninsula and
Greater Williamsburg
Building Partner

Get involved today, visit
www.MorganJamesBuilds.com.

To My Husband
Steven

To My Beautiful Children
Joshua and Ariel

To all of the women who have struggled in the
darkness without the benefit of enlightenment

Table of Contents

Surviving the Emotional Turbulence of the Fifth Decade

Jerilynn C. Prior BA, MD, FRCPC,

Professor of Endocrinology, Director of the Centre
for Menstrual Cycle and Ovulation Research
University of British Columbia and
Vancouver Coastal Health Research Institute

*O*ut of the blue, Deborah Wagner, a psychologist from New Jersey, emailed asking to use a table I created about the "Phases of Perimenopause"[1] in her new book, *The Fifth Decade—Is it Just My Life or is it Perimenopause?* I well remember creating that table, scribbling on lined yellow paper at my breakfast nook in the wee hours—at the time I had the elated feeling that my integration was creative and important. That table was part of a provocative review confirming the new idea that estrogen levels rise rather than drop in

---

1   Prior, J.C. (1998). Perimenopause: The complex endocrinology of the menopausal transition. *Endocrine Reviews*, 19:397-428.

perimenopause and trying to figure out how these changes relate to women's experiences. The table revealed, what I believed but didn't dare yet spell out, that perimenopause begins, not when cycles "get funny" but when *experiences* have changed.[2] Higher estrogen (and lower progesterone) levels are unique, and experience changes are new—thus even with bang-on regular periods, a new name is needed: *perimenopause.*

I was gratified that my integration of perimenopausal hormonal swings with the physical and emotional changes of midlife caught Dr. Wagner's eye. Of course she could reprint this table! But please use a more recent, refined version.[3]

I soon learned that Dr. Wagner is as committed as I am to making accurate perimenopause information available to the many perplexed and frustrated midlife women. On that basis I agreed to read her book and write this Foreword. I admit that I was initially apprehensive that she, as others have, would take the equally wrong approaches of blaming women's "midlife madness" on "estrogen deficiency" or attributing it solely to distress over aging as people who rely on sexual allure for our value in the social hierarchy. Instead, Dr. Wagner has done an excellent job of balancing individual personality traits, past and present life experiences, lack of cogent, helpful midlife transition information and the hormonal chaos of perimenopause, **all** of which contribute to perimenopausal "Turbulence."

Having read it, I believe that *The Fifth Decade* will be a life-saver for the many young-looking women in their late thirties and forties who, besides being on an emotional and physiological rollercoaster, are wrongly told that dropping estrogen levels are responsible for

---

2 Prior, J.C. (2005). Clearing confusion about perimenopause. B.C.M.J., 47(10): 534-8.

3 Prior, J.C. (2002). The ageing female reproductive axis II: ovulatory changes with perimenopause. In: Chadwick DJ, Goode JA, editors. Endocrine Facets of Ageing. 242 ed. Chichester, UK: John Wiley and Sons Ltd., 172-86.

their misery. What helps most of all, is to know, that they, in Dr. Wagner's terms, will move from "Turbulence" to eventual "Quietude" as they survive perimenopause and thrive in a calmer, gentler menopause.[4]

I recall so well those days in my late 40s when, though my periods were regular, I was totally miserable. I cried during my three kilometer walk up hill through parks and by single family homes to the Osteoporosis Clinic of which I was then director. Although a hormone expert, I didn't know why I was falling apart. It was worse because, whatever was making me miserable, I had to hide it from my patients and colleagues. At the clinic I found an isolated washroom in which to blow my nose and wash my face—if asked, I bravely grinned and blamed my swollen eyes on "bad allergies."

The good news is that *The Fifth Decade* amazingly integrates midlife mind and body and much, much more. Many social scientists past and present seem allergic to anything of the body[5,6] and want to blame all on an "empty nest," or loss of fertility and youth, and sexual allure or fear of aging. An alternative is to blame estrogen deficiency for everything.[7] However, making a connection, as this book does, between the truly higher and swinging levels of estrogens of perimenopause and women's midlife emotions, is a major advance for women.

I am also astonished and gratified that Dr. Wagner considers ***progesterone to be the "feel good hormone."*** Even I, who believe strongly in the power of progesterone, would not be so baldly positive. I had come to believe, however, in progesterone's important role in women's health after 30 years of research on its functions within regular cycles, in perimenopause and in menopause.

---

4   Prior, J.C. (2006). Perimenopause lost—reframing the end of menstruation. Journal of Reproductive and Infant Psychology. 24(4):323-35.

5   Sheehy, G. (1992). The Silent Passage. New York: Random House.

6   Page, L. (1993). Menopause and emotions: making sense of your feelings when your feelings make no sense. 1ed. Vancouver: Primavera Press.

7   Wilson, R.A. (1966). Feminine Forever. New York: M. Evans & Co., Inc.

For example, Centre for Menstrual Cycle and Ovulation Research *(www.cemcor.ubc.ca)* studies show that bone loss occurs when premenopausal women have silent lack of ovulation and lower levels of progesterone, this despite normal estrogen levels and regular cycles.[8, 9] In perimenopause, the decreasing progesterone levels (with higher swinging estrogens) increase the heavy flow, weight gain and sore breasts; but oral micronized progesterone treatment is found to be highly effective for hot flushes and night sweats in menopausal women.[10] By contrast, many of my colleagues blame progesterone for everything bad that women experience—depression, bloating, breast cancer and heart attacks. After all, in our culture it is "estrogen (that) makes a girl, a girl!" By contrast, I *say*, "Progesterone with estrogen makes a girl, a woman!"[11]

While you read, *The Fifth Decade* be prepared to giggle or laugh out loud as Wagner recounts women finding lost keys snuggled with the milk in the fridge, waking with "pjs" inside out or discovering they have poured orange juice rather than cream into their coffee! Stories pepper this book. Stories that feel authentic, of women's lives, social situations and emotional distresses. Most thoughtful and important of all, Wagner describes four perimenopausal emotional phases with the last one being "Quietude." This is much like I envision "estrogen's storm season"[12]

---

8 Prior, J.C., Vigna, Y.M., Schechter, M.T., & Burgess, A.E. (1990). Spinal bone loss and ovulatory disturbances. NEJM, 323:1221-7.

9 Bedford, J.L., Prior, J.C., & Barr, S.I. (2010). A prospective exploration of cognitive dietary restraint, subclinical ovulatory disturbances, cortisol and change in bone density over two years in healthy young women. JCEM, 95:3291-9.

10 Prior, J.C. & Hitchcock, C.L. (2010). Progesterone for vasomotor symptoms: A 12-week randomized, masked placebo-controlled trial in healthy, normal-weight women 1-10 years since final menstrual flow. Endocrine Reviews, 31(3), S51. Ref Type: Abstract.

11 Baxter S., Prior, J.C. (2009). The Estrogen Errors: Why Progesterone is Better For Women's Health. Westport: Praeger Publishers.

12 Prior, J.C. (2007). Estrogen's Storm Season—Stories of Perimenopause. Vancouver, BC: CeMCOR. (2005).

of perimenopause eventually becoming the safe and quiet harbor of menopause.

Dr. Wagner illustrates the complex interplay of personality, past life experiences, present hormonal chaos and current social situations with midlife women's vivid dreams of pregnancy and other dreams. Through these dreams and how they fit into women's stories, we perceive that dreams involve important emotional work. Through this book, we begin to understand and learn to better deal with the ***emotional transition*** of perimenopause to which the transient hormonal chaos of midlife is strongly related.

Acknowledgements

While only my name appears as the author of this book, there are many who have contributed to its creation. I am grateful for the countless scientists and researchers whose works are referenced in this book--works that have laid the foundation for the emerging wisdom about women in perimenopause.

There are a number of individuals who have been instrumental in helping me bring this book to fruition. I thank my agent, Michael Ebeling, who had enough faith in my project to open the doors to my publisher.

I am deeply appreciative of the countless hours spent by Dale Pozzi, a brilliant editor, who helped me get this project off the ground. I also thank Sharyn Lustig for her comments and advice.

I am so grateful to my friend and advisor, Jeffrey Schantz, for stepping out of his "comfort zone" to guide me through some difficult decisions.

My appreciation goes to Jerilynn Prior, M.D. for all she has provided to expanding the knowledge base of perimenopause and for her contributions to this book.

I give my heartiest gratitude to my family. Each contributed in their own unique way to the completion of this book. I owe my son, Joshua Grundleger, who tirelessly critiqued and polished every word of this book, a debt of gratitude. My husband, Steven Grundleger, never failed to supply an encouraging word, along with all of the technological savvy I could ever wish for. My daughter, Ariel Grundleger, always ready with a hug when this project seemed daunting, got me through some very frustrating moments. Alexandra Grundleger diligently worked to give me a fresh perspective. I thank Barbara and Albert Wagner for their support and encouragement and Lillian Levine who always said I could do this.

Prologue

When I was in graduate school studying life-span developmental psychology, we learned about changes in morality, intelligence and familial roles. There was little to no focus on women, as being so very different from men. On the contrary, that was an era when our culture seemed to be trying to collapse the differences between men and women in order to equalize the sexes. This did a great disservice to women as we embarked on a mission of denying the unique qualities and needs that we have as women. In my clinical practice as a psychologist, I have treated people from age two to 80, men, women, couples and families. One group has stood out as having unique needs that were barely understood; perimenopausal women.

Perimenopause is the time in a woman's life that precedes menopause typically by five to ten years. This is a period in which a woman's physiology and emotions are shifting significantly and are typically not well understood by the medical and psychological communities. Although there is a wealth of literature and understanding about menopause, the study of perimenopause as a separate entity is only just evolving to be explored and understood.

In my clinical practice I have seen women in the perimenopausal stage of life, typically aged between forty and fifty, struggling with a host of emotional issues that are not typical of other age ranges. The problems they struggle with are somewhat unique to this stage of life and often seem to baffle the women, themselves. They find their prior methods of coping or dealing with difficulties no longer work for them.

This is often a stage in women's lives marked by drastic relationship and role changes. In our culture, women frequently are preparing to end their roles as active parents as their children start college or jobs and become independent financially and/or emotionally. This not only impacts how women view themselves but also affects how husband and wife relate to one another. Often, there are tremendous upheavals in spousal or partner relationships that seem to have come out of nowhere. Partners are confused as to why suddenly they have relationship problems and prior issues seem to worsen. These emotional issues are interwoven with a host of physiological changes.

Women experience changes in their bodies, including shifts in metabolism, ability to get restful sleep, menstrual cycle changes and reduced stamina. Often this creates a spiral in which physiological changes and psychological changes begin to negatively impact the other, such that a woman finds it difficult to "feel herself."

Before a woman can successfully emerge from this difficult but confusing phase of life, she must first understand what is happening to her, and why. *The Fifth Decade* will focus on how the physiological changes of perimenopause become wrapped up with psychological and emotional changes and what women can do to untangle, and hence proceed through them.

Perimenopause is the stage in a woman's life immediately prior to menopause. It can last from two to ten years before menstruation stops entirely. For some women, perimenopause is relatively uneventful, bringing change but not to a disruptive level. For other women, perimenopausal changes can be intense enough to cause significant distress. Common symptoms are the interruption of restful sleep, diminishing sexual interest, shifting moods and a reduced sense of wellbeing. The good news is that the instability does diminish over time. I have identified four psychological stages of perimenopause through which most women will pass: Stage I, Perimenopausal Initiation, Stage II, Emotional Disruption, Stage III Turbulence and Stage IV, Quietude.

In the pages that follow, I will help women recognize the emotional and physiological challenges they can expect to experience during the volatile years of perimenopause. While some women have learned that they can expect to feel angry and aggressive in the years before their periods end, they are often unaware that a great many other emotional changes—such as a changing libido, a lessened ability to empathize with others, exhaustion, depression, a sense of isolation and lack of connection with trusted friends and associates—are actually attributable to the fluctuations occurring during perimenopause.

During this window, the relationships that women build throughout their lives can become jeopardized. As a therapist, I have come to understand that this period of change is extremely confusing and disruptive for women and those closest to them. I have also come to recognize that it helps significantly to be able to put a name and a reason to the chaos. It is important to understand that when a woman's body enters perimenopause, the regular cycling of hormones that she has been accustomed to since puberty undergoes a change. An irregular pattern of hormonal fluctuations, beginning with a significant rise in levels of estrogen and ending with a gradual overall decrease in estrogen and progesterone is activated.

Before beginning our discussion, I provide an overview of key physiological factors that play an important role in the emotional and other changes that occur during perimenopause. I will refer to these in the following chapters and explain the role they play in psychological symptomology. These factors will include:

FSH and LH

When a woman's body enters perimenopause the regular cycling of hormones to which she has been accustomed since puberty begins to undergo a change. Although all of the hormones: estrogen, progesterone, follicle stimulating hormone (FSH) and luteinizing hormone (LH) continue to cycle, the patterns become unbalanced. This is often when emotional trouble begins.

Estrogen is the hormone responsible for maturation and development of the female sex organs and secondary sexual characteristics. Estrogen is also responsible for cell growth, increasing the number of cells found in several centers of the brain and body, determining our functioning. It is estrogen that is responsible for the greater experience of physical pain and "gut feelings" in women relative to men.

Throughout the menstrual cycle, estrogen is responsible for a multitude of symptoms including headaches, water retention, increased depression and an imbalance of blood sugar. It is instrumental in affecting the cyclic variations in cognition and impacting the sex drive. Estrogen also plays a role in stabilizing fluctuating moods.

Progesterone

Progesterone receptors are present throughout the entire body. Its effects are present in every location in which there is a receptor. Progesterone is a precursor in the production of other hormones, including estrogen, testosterone and cortisol. It helps maintain healthy thyroid function, promotes healthy bone density, utilizes body fat for fuel, and is indicated in the prevention of breast, ovarian and uterine cancers.

Progesterone also helps to stabilize blood sugar levels, fight heart disease by maintaining proper blood clotting, increase sex drive, and, of course, is a major player in procreation. One of the more important functions of progesterone is that it counteracts many of the unpleasant effects of estrogen. Progesterone levels decline over the course of perimenopause.

Sex Hormones in Puberty

Female hormones are responsible for changes to the brain and its neuro-hormones (hormones secreted by the body or nervous system that have an effect on the nervous system) that begin in puberty. Behaviors, including intimacy and aggression, evolve and intensify with the production of large amounts of estrogen and progesterone during puberty. These hormones begin to cycle monthly with fluctuations on a daily and/or weekly basis. During the second and third weeks of the menstrual cycle, androgen levels peak. Females with low androgen levels generally have a weaker sex drive and are less aggressive.

Premenstrual Syndrome (PMS)

PMS encompasses a host of physiological and psychological changes in the two weeks prior to menstruation and occasionally a couple of days into menstruation. When a woman experiences PMS, her estrogen levels increase while progesterone levels are insufficient to balance the estrogen.

Cortisol

One of the adrenal hormones, cortisol is commonly referred to as the "stress hormone." When a woman is under continued, abundant stress, her adrenal glands begin to secrete an excess of cortisol.

Thyroid Hormones

The prevalence of thyroid disorders increases dramatically in women in their forties and fifties. With the onset of perimenopause, women with or without prior thyroid illness may have a more difficult time managing their thyroid hormone levels. In both cases we may see a significant rise in depression and anxiety as a result of an inadequately functioning metabolism and endocrine system.

Menstrual Changes in Perimenopause

There are a number of typical patterns in which menstruation changes at the onset of perimenopause. The menstrual cycle can become irregular in terms of onset, duration and/or flow. The length of a cycle may initially shorten to as few as two weeks and later double from the premenopausal twenty-eight days to a late perimenopausal cycle of fifty-eight days and longer. Toward the end of perimenopause, several months will pass between periods. Women are not considered to have reached menopause until they have gone one full year without having a period.

Part I

THE PHYSIOLOGICAL UNDERPINNINGS OF THE PSYCHOLOGY OF PERIMENOPAUSE

This section will give an overview of the hormonal patterns before and during perimenopause and a sense of how these hormonal changes affect women physically. Unbelievably, it was not until 2001 that perimenopause was officially defined as a distinct phenomenon, differing from menopause![1] Typically, perimenopause starts when a woman is in her forties, but may begin as early as the mid-thirties. The median age for the beginning of perimenopause is between forty-five and forty-seven years of age,[2] and menopause occurs at an average age of 51.3 years.[3]

The changing pattern of menstruation is what initially alerts women to their entry into perimenopause. The cycle begins to change in terms of duration of menses or time in between periods. As one gets closer to menopause, entire periods are skipped. The fundamental event that takes place during and after perimenopause is that a woman's reproductive ability diminishes until it eventually ceases. The notable effect this may have on women psychologically will be explored later. Understanding the challenges and changes that surface during perimenopause help women negotiate this difficult transition.

Jerilynn Prior, a leading perimenopause researcher, sectioned the perimenopausal transition into five phases.[4] Her phases help identify the physiological changes women experience as they progress through perimenopause (Table 0-1). Phase A is defined by intermittently high estradiol (a type of estrogen) levels with symptoms of weight gain, migraines and heavy menstrual flow. Periods are still regular, with normal ovulation but there are increased symptoms of PMS: breast tenderness, bloating and mood swings. The follicular phase of the menstrual cycle shortens, as does the menstrual period. Women may experience their first early morning night sweats.

During Phase B, menstrual cycles are still somewhat regular but ovulation is no longer predictable, with some cycles being anovulatory (without ovulation). PMS continues to worsen and vasomotor symptoms increase just prior to menstruation. Additionally, follicle stimulating hormone (FSH) begins to fluctuate to a higher level during the early follicular phase.

Phase C is characterized by increasing variability in the duration, flow and regularity of periods. Vasomotor symptoms begin to appear, primarily during the daytime hours but are not yet too problematic. Estradiol levels show wide variability, from extremely high, to normal or low, and FSH levels begin to show a more regular elevation.

In Phase D, menstruation begins to slow down in frequency, duration and flow. There are occasional cycles that may be particularly troublesome in terms of symptoms, usually after there has been a skipped period or a long delay since the prior one. More than 50 percent of cycles are anovulatory, creating a significant deficit of progesterone. Vasomotor symptoms are gaining strength and FSH is consistently elevated, as is leutenizing hormone (LH).

Phase E is the beginning of the end. Vasomotor symptoms intensify to an uncomfortable degree but symptoms of PMS lessen. There may occasionally be a pseudo-PMS, that is, premenstrual symptoms with no subsequent menstruation. This phase of perimenopause begins with the last menstrual period and lasts for one year until menopause has been established. FSH and LH are high, while estrogen levels are low.

These five phases are not necessarily linear and may overlap at some points. Some women may oscillate between two phases, or even three before settling in to one. It is helpful, however to keep this progression of phases in mind as we learn more about the specifics of the perimeno-pausal changes. The terminology and concepts used may be unfamiliar, but will be explained in more depth as we proceed.

Table 0-1
Proposed Phases of the Perimenopause: Clinical and Hormonal Characteristics[5]

	Phase A	Phase B	Phase C	Phase D	Phase E
Duration	2–6 months		1–2 yr	1–2 yr	1 yr
Menstrual cycles	Regular, ovulatory shorter cycles, short follicular phases	Regular, often ovulatory disturbances	Irregular, alternate short and long cycles, ovulation less than 50%		Amenorrhea
Flow	Increased or the same	Increased	↑↑ or less, often alternating	Spotting alternating with flooding	None
Menstrual cycle-related symptoms	↑PMS ↑Dysmenorrhea, breast symptoms, exacerbation of headaches and migraines	↑↑PMS, intermittent dysmenorrhea	Less PMS but erratic, menstrual-type cramps may occur any time	No predictable symptoms, menstrual-like cramps in a few women, anytime	Few or confusing without subsequent flow

Vasomotor symptoms	First onset, cyclic before flow or midcycle (very often in the early morning)	Cyclic still during or at the end of sleep	Still cyclic, but less predictable, onset in daytime	Erratic, more persistent in long cycles	May become consistent daily, or decrease
Hormonal characteristics	Normal FSH, ↑E_2 short follicular phases, LH normal, ? inhibin low	↑FSH intermittent, ↑E_2 at flow for some nonovulatory cycles, LH normal, ? inhibin low	Normal alternating with high E_2 ↑FSH persistently, ↑LH occasionally, ? inhibin low	↑FSH, ↑LH, E_2 normal except intermittent prolonged high levels, inhibin low	↑↑FSH, ↑↑LH Normal or low E_2, but intermittent low or high levels, below assay inhibin sensitivity

PMS, Premenstrual symptoms; E_2, estradiol;

↑ moderately increased; ↑↑ very high.

While the first signal a woman often notices on her entry into perimenopause is the change in menses, it is not the first effect of perimenopause. I hope to bring awareness to women that the first sign is more typically a shift in emotions, moods and a way of engaging with the world. This psychological change is the signal that is not usually noticed as a sign of perimenopause until much later, often once the change in emotionality is of disruptive proportions.

Although Part I of this book focuses on the physiology of perimenopause and Part II on the psychology of perimenopause, I want to make it very clear that these two aspects of perimenopause are interactional components that are bidirectional, each one influencing the other. The precise process of how the physiology and psychology in a perimenopausal woman mutually affect one another is only just beginning to be understood.

Chapter One

Changing Hormones Equals Changing Emotions

It was Monday morning and Sari awoke to the sound of her alarm clock. Her husband, Sam, walked over to the bed, gave her a hug and asked her to join him for breakfast, which was almost ready in the kitchen. He was happy and smiling and ready to start the week. Sari shook her head, fighting the tears that were about to spill over. She did not have the heart to bring Sam down again. When Sam left to have his breakfast, Sari dragged herself into the shower. As the hot water poured over her, she allowed the tears to flow, as she had done so many times before. For the hundredth, if not the thousandth time, Sari searched her heart and her mind for what could possibly be so wrong to make her feel this way. With a loving husband, happy healthy children, financial security and a job she loved, why now, was she so miserable?

When a woman's body enters perimenopause the regular cycling of hormones that she has been accustomed to since puberty begins to undergo a change. An irregular pattern of hormonal fluctuations is activated, beginning with a significant rise in levels of estrogen and ending with a gradual decrease in estrogen and progesterone.[6] Although all of the hormones, estrogen, progesterone, follicle stimulating hormone (FSH) and luteinizing hormone (LH) are still cycling, the patterns of the cycle begin to become unbalanced. This is often when the emotional struggles begin.

Before a woman enters perimenopause, approximately a week after menstruation has begun, low estrogen levels signal FSH to stimulate the ovarian follicles to maturity. One prevailing follicle matures and begins secreting large quantities of estrogen. This in turn, shuts down further production of FSH and stimulates the release of LH, a signal of imminent ovulation. Ovulation is the process by which the follicle ruptures and the egg is released. The ruptured follicle, the corpus luteum, now begins to secrete large quantities of progesterone in preparation for a potential pregnancy. When no pregnancy occurs, the corpus luteum depletes its store of hormones, which results in a lowering of estrogen and progesterone. The lining of the uterus prepares for shedding and menstruation begins along with a new cycle.

When women are in their late thirties, their ovaries begin to accelerate the ripening and loss of follicles every month. Eventually, the number of follicles available for ovulation diminishes until there are none left. This is the body's way of discarding old, potentially defective eggs. FSH increases as it did before, but in the forty-something perimenopausal woman the follicles are no longer as sensitive to the effects of FSH. FSH is knocking on the follicle door, but no one is answering. With the lowered sensitivity to FSH and the highly variable amount of estrogen that is secreted, FSH production is not suppressed. In early perimenopause when estrogen levels may be even higher than in the premenopausal woman, FSH levels are still on the rise (when, in fact, they should be falling).[7] The problem this creates is that with elevated FSH levels, LH is not signaled for secretion. Without LH no follicle matures, no follicle is ruptured, no egg is released, there is no corpus luteum and progesterone production is not signaled. This is the process by which women begin having anovulatory cycles in perimenopause[8] and the start of the emotional ups and downs that we saw in Sari.

These changes in the menstrual cycle do not follow a linear pattern, and that makes this period a very trying one. A woman may have months of normal cycles followed by a stretch of irregular cycles. Some women have a pattern of one month normal, and the next irregular but any type of pattern is possible. In one study on perimenopausal women, 100 different patterns of menstrual flow and cycles were documented in 300 women![9] This irregular releasing of the hormones creates the variability in the menstrual cycles causing the physiological and psychological effects of perimenopause. As we will learn in the coming chapters, estrogen and progesterone have powerful effects on mood. When estrogen levels plummet, women will experience anxiety, especially if progesterone levels are low or declining with the estrogen. With estrogen levels bouncing around, as they do in perimenopause, a woman's mood, or ability to tolerate stressful events changes in accordance with those estrogen level changes.

When no progesterone is produced in the anovulatory cycles, there is an insufficient amount of progesterone in comparison to the amount of estrogen. This creates a situation called "estrogen dominance." As we will learn, balance among hormones is key to feelings of wellbeing. Estrogen dominance in combination with excess FSH and the elevation of estrogen in the follicular phase of the menstrual cycle are all major culprits in the emotional distress of perimenopause.[10, 11]

Progesterone is the "feel good" hormone. In pregnancy, it is the abundance of progesterone that leaves women with a peaceful, calm and radiant emotional experience. In perimenopause when progesterone is in short supply and estrogen levels are erratic, women are inclined to feel that the protective barriers between their emotional stability and the outside world are dangerously fragile.

The changing hormone levels are all very clinical and scientific but what is important to understand is how estrogen and progesterone affect how we feel and how we behave. We will begin to understand Sari's changes in mood as we learn more about the physiological and social psychological challenges that Sari will experience as she passes through perimenopause on her way to menopause.

Chapter Two

Almighty Estrogen

$\mathcal{P}$uberty is a young woman's first experience with a huge rise in estrogen levels. Valerie, at 11 years old was on the cusp of puberty. Her ovaries began secreting large amounts of estrogen. This initiated the maturation and development of her female sex organs and secondary sexual characteristics. Valerie began to experience breast development and growth of hair in the pubic area and in her armpits. Her figure began changing with the widening of her hips and slimming of her waist. What Valerie was unaware of, was that the estrogen was also preparing her uterus to begin menstruation and eventually to be ready for pregnancy. Valerie had yet to learn that this new influx of estrogen was at least partially responsible for the cycling symptoms of breast tenderness, bloating and moodiness that were soon to become a powerful disruption to the simple easy emotions of childhood.

Estrogen's influence in the body is enormously powerful. It affects cell growth in the body and in the brain. It is the hormone implicated in women's ability to tolerate more physical pain than men and the development of the notorious and very real "women's intuition." Researchers believe this is due to the greater number of cells in specific areas of the brain that track bodily sensations.

During the stage of infantile puberty, a period that lasts from birth until two years of age, the female infant's ovaries produce a large quantity of estrogen, comparable to the levels found in adults. This estrogen not only prepares the ovaries for later reproductive capabilities but also has a major impact on the development of the brain. Neurons grow and develop, creating brain circuits with a specifically female bias. The female brain, bathing in estrogen, becomes more developed in the areas of observation and communication, giving women unique capabilities in these areas.[12]

As Valerie progresses through puberty and estrogen begins to change the structure of her brain, she will become more intuitive, nurturing and caring. Research shows that these areas of the brain are more highly developed in females as a result of the high estrogen levels. Practically speaking, this leaves a female more capable of reading facial expressions, of hearing emotional nuance in vocalizations, of interpreting and responding to "body language" or unspoken cues in others. When Valerie is mingling with her other adolescent girlfriends, they will all automatically utilize these new skills to communicate and understand each other. These attributes allow for greater socialization between girls along with an inclination to create a community with others.[13]

Estrogen is a bit more complex than it seems. "Estrogen" is actually a term that is used to represent the three different types of estrogen that exist in the human body. The first estrogen, estrone, makes up about 10 to 20 percent of circulating estrogens before menopause. After menopause, estrone becomes the principal estrogen in the body since the levels of estrone drop off less than the levels of the other estrogens.[14,15] There is a notable dearth of information on estrone and emotion but some obscure data suggests that estrone levels are extremely reactive to stress. Stressful situations will depress estrone levels for several days before there is a rebounding to normal levels.[16]

The second estrogen, estradiol, makes up another 10 to 20 percent of the circulating estrogens before menopause. Estradiol is the estrogen we most often associate with the feminine characteristics of estrogen. This is the type of estrogen that gave Valerie mature egg-bearing follicles, her developed breasts and fertile ovaries and uterus. Until recently it was believed that perimenopause was the opposite of puberty-that in puberty estradiol steadily increased, with the onset of perimenopause it steadily decreased.

Current research[17] has shown the opposite of what was believed for generations. Early in perimenopause estradiol levels actually increase significantly. Estradiol levels in the follicular phase of the menstrual cycle in perimenopausal women exceed the estradiol levels in the same phase of the menstrual cycle in premenopausal woman. These shifting levels of estradiol are believed to be responsible for many of the emotional difficulties in early perimenopause.[18] When estradiol levels begin to fall, it is the reduction of estradiol that accounts for the increase in anxiety and depression[19, 20] during perimenopause. Supporting research has shown an improvement in depressive symptoms when perimenopausal women were supplemented with estradiol.[21]

One other significant function of estradiol is that it is the estrogen most influential in evoking maternal behaviors. This is the estrogen that compels women to nurture. When women are of childbearing age it is critical to have an ample amount of estradiol in order to facilitate mothering. Do we need as much of this hormone once we are past childbearing? We will explore later the implications of the dramatic decrease in this estrogen at the end of perimenopause and how it affects nurturing behaviors.

The third estrogen is estriol. Estriol, the weakest estrogen, accounts for 60 to 80 percent of the circulating estrogens. Estriol is the only estrogen that has anticancer properties. The other main function of estriol is that when abundant, it has positive effects on the urogenital tissues. As it declines with perimenopause, it contributes to the thinning of these tissues which not only causes physical discomfort, but also indirectly negatively influences mood.

Often women are not able to enjoy sex because it has become painful due to inadequate vaginal lubrication from decreasing estriol. This may introduce or augment emotional challenges already present from shifting hormones. Relief of these symptoms has been accomplished by using a topical estriol cream.[22] Estriol, similar to estrone, has been found to decrease in response to stressful stimuli.[23] We can begin to see the interactive effects of our female hormones and our moods. When stress suppresses the very hormones women need to manage stress, they are truly challenged!

Chapter Three
Puberty and PMS: Emotional Hostage Takers

Puberty

Perimenopause has been equated with two, perhaps more familiar, difficult hormonal events in women's lives: puberty and premenstrual syndrome (PMS). Puberty is the first time in a female's life that her brain is flooded with estrogen and progesterone, produced by the ovaries. These hormones begin to cycle monthly with fluctuations on a daily and or weekly basis. As Louann Brizendine, a neuropsychiatrist who specializes in the workings of the female brain explains, "The rising tide of estrogen and progesterone starts to fuel many circuits in the teen girl's brain that were laid down in fetal life. These new hormonal surges assure that all of her female-specific brain circuits will become even more sensitive to emotional nuance."[24] This is when we see adolescents, like Valerie, becoming highly reactive to the slightest intimation of emotion. Valerie will be brought to tears over a sad story of a homeless kitten or have fits of rage because a parent reminds her of her curfew in front of her friends. Every day she will have new issues with her friends. Parents will find it next to impossible to keep up with all of the "drama."

Progesterone and estrogen directly affect many parts of the brain, in particular the areas for memory and learning, the area responsible for emotions, and the brain's ability to negotiate stress, which varies with the changing hormonal levels.

As females reach puberty, their overall responsivity to stress intensifies from what it was prior to puberty and shows an increase in comparison to male responsivity to stress. The type of events that stress an adolescent female becomes more specific, for instance, relationship conflicts are the more threatening issues to an adolescent female compared to a male who is more stressed by authority challenges than social conflict.[25] Anyone who knows an adolescent female is familiar with how sensitive girls at this age are to social stresses. The positive side is that the female brain that is exposed to estrogen is compelled to respond with nurturing behaviors to stressful stimuli. This will be a more reliable response once the volatility of rapidly shifting pubescent hormones has quieted down.

Puberty brings with it another hormonal surge, that of the androgens. Testosterone, DHEA and androstenedione are the three main androgens that begin to increase in puberty, peaking at nineteen years of age. While testosterone and DHEA are associated with sexual interest, androstenedione is associated with aggressiveness. The second and third weeks of the menstrual cycle see the androgen levels peak. Females with low androgen levels generally have a weaker sex drive and are less aggressive. Here again, we see how influential hormones are on human behavior. Now we can begin to understand why our pubescent girls are such whirling forces of emotional confusion. One moment they are loving and nurturing, while the next they are aggressive, sarcastic or socially "phobic" and the next are sexy little vamps!

To complicate matters further, another significant development at puberty is the activation of oxytocin and dopamine by ovarian estrogen.

Oxytocin is a neurohormone in females that is involved with human intimacy. It evokes and is evoked by intimate behaviors. When estrogen is at its highest in the middle of the menstrual cycle so are oxytocin and dopamine (a neurochemical that stimulates the pleasure centers in the brain and creates a sense of wellbeing). Intimate behaviors, including verbal intimacy, physical intimacy, sexual intimacy and other bonding behaviors are being chemically encouraged by this increase in oxytocin and dopamine.[26] With the influx of oxytocin, our little Valerie becomes the wonderful girl we love to hug.

Understanding the evolution of the female hormones and their effects on the brain and neurohormones in puberty is helpful in understanding the challenges of perimenopause. As we see certain behaviors evolve with the influx of estrogen and progesterone into the body in large amounts at puberty, we can appreciate how some of these same behaviors and emotions are affected in the opposite direction as the hormones begin to ebb later in life in perimenopause. We can also begin to understand what actions we can take to stimulate or replace some of the hormones that are being reduced in perimenopause and why so many of our emotions and preferences feel so alien to us in this transition.

PMS

PMS is a result of a number of physiological and psychological changes in the two weeks prior to menstruation and occasionally lasting a couple of days into menstruation. Severe PMS affects up to five percent of all premenopausal women while mild PMS affects a third of all premenopausal women. Unfortunately, it is not commonly understood that PMS severity increases as women enter perimenopause. The unpleasant physical sensations of PMS that women experience include bloating, food cravings, headaches, loss of energy, breast tenderness, backache and abdominal cramps. The psychological symptoms of PMS typically include depression, anxiety, moodiness, feelings of fatigue, inability to concentrate, panic attacks and irritability.

What is happening on a hormonal level when a woman is experiencing PMS is her estrogen levels are increasing while her progesterone levels are low. Unfortunately, this may occur even when the progesterone levels are elevated if a woman is stressed. This is because levels of cortisol, an adrenal hormone involved in stress reactions, are increased, blocking the progesterone receptors' ability to accept the progesterone. So, progesterone is trying to get in to exert its calming effects, but cortisol is blocking the way. Once again we can see how stress can mitigate the beneficial properties of hormones.

The menstrual cycle is a much "bigger deal" than most people realize. It is quite a bit more than having a few more or less hormones and then a period. Female hormones create actual changes in the brain structure in the first two weeks of the menstrual cycle. A part of the brain called the hippocampus grows by 25 percent due to the increase in estrogen. The hippocampus is extremely sensitive to estrogen and is responsible for verbal processing and verbal memory. This better functioning brain thinks more clearly and quickly and has a better memory. This is the best time in the menstrual cycle to go for that job interview or take that important exam.

Mid-cycle, at ovulation, progesterone is secreted and these new brain connections are destroyed, resulting in the slowing of those same brain functions, while simultaneously leaving a calming effect.

In the last days of the menstrual cycle, progesterone production shuts down and the resulting effect is an anxious and irritable brain that has lost the soothing elements of the progesterone. The psychological effects of this brain irritability leave women feeling moody, depressed, anxious, explosive and weepy.

We can now understand why there is such a difference between the emotional response patterns of the first and second halves of a woman's menstrual cycle. In the first two weeks, with high estrogen levels, she will be more socially engaged and relaxed. Midcycle, high progesterone leaves her feeling calm and happy. As the hormones shift to lower estrogen, and the progesterone begins falling off in the second two weeks, she will become more anxious, irritable and reclusive. In more severe PMS, mood swings often deteriorate into uncontrollable behaviors such as rage and clinical depression.

This latter pattern is more characteristic of women in perimenopause who experience a worsening of the symptoms of PMS. This is in addition to a host of other symptoms that develop as perimenopause progresses. The fluctuations of the hormones in the two weeks before menstruation become intensified, creating an increase in hormone related mood symptoms. Since both progesterone and cortisol compete for the same receptors in cells, an excess of cortisol secretion as a result of stress can be a direct cause of estrogen dominance, a major contributor to the symptoms of perimenopause, similar to how progesterone and cortisol battle during PMS.

Chapter Four

Navigating the Storm

*I*t is common for people who do not have an understanding of what is happening in their bodies to initially worry about and eventually fear what may be wrong with them. I have worked with many individuals who experience physiological changes and who immediately ponder the worst-case scenario. This was the case with one woman whose perimenopausal forgetfulness had her convinced she had a brain tumor. Such fear occasionally inhibits the individual from seeking medical attention because they begin to dread receiving "bad news" This not only increases the risk of suffering from anxiety, but can also lead to depressive symptoms.

In perimenopause, there is a wide range of physiological symptoms that can arouse significant concern if not understood. It is also more likely that a woman in perimenopause will experience an anxious or depressed state simply because of the shifting hormones. This chapter provides an overview of some of the many physiological changes that evolve throughout perimenopause so that women can feel comfortable with the normal changes happening in their bodies.

PMS

As women get older, it becomes more and more difficult to differentiate between the symptoms of PMS and those of perimenopause. Ovarian changes often begin when women are in their thirties and may present as worsening PMS symptoms. The late thirties into the forties is the age range when women report the worst PMS symptoms. The major difference between the very similar symptoms of PMS and perimenopause is that in PMS the symptoms show an abrupt improvement with the onset of menses. This is not so with perimenopause, when symptoms may carry well into the menstrual cycle.

Changes in Menstruation

As long as her periods are regular, a woman may believe she is not yet in perimenopause. This is not necessarily the case. Once her periods do become irregular, this is an indication she has begun perimenopause. There are a number of common ways in which menstruation may change. The menstrual cycle can become irregular in terms of onset, duration and/or flow. Some women, like Linda, find their cycles have become elongated, waiting more than a month between periods. Others find their cycles becoming shorter, with periods coming every two to three weeks. Still others find an erratic or changeable pattern of some cycles being long while others are short. Cycle length can vary by more than a week early in perimenopause.

In middle to late perimenopause the irregularity in cycle length tends to form a pattern of shorter cycles followed by longer cycles, with an increasing number of days between cycles. Late in the menopausal transition, women's cycles lengthen to the point where periods are skipped altogether. The length of a cycle will double from the premenopausal twenty-eight days to a late perimenopausal cycle of fifty-eight days or longer.[27] Eventually, several months will pass between periods. Women are not considered to have completed menopause until they have gone one full year without having a period.

Menstrual flow will also change with the onset of perimenopause. Some women will experience minor changes while others will experience drastic changes in the heaviness of their menstrual flow. Early in perimenopause more women report having a heavier flow, sometimes extraordinarily heavy, to the point of "flooding," a situation in which the blood flow is so heavy, it will soak through pads and clothing in a short period of time.

Tara's Story

Tara, a medical health professional in her late forties began to notice changes in her menstrual cycle. First her periods began to come less frequently, the time between periods stretching to five or six weeks. This lasted for a period of about six months. Then her cycles began to shorten to about three weeks between periods. To Tara's shock, one day, while with a patient, Tara felt a wetness; she excused herself and went to the ladies' room. She discovered her period blood her soaked through her napkin, had run down her legs and into her shoes.

This was Tara's concrete and undeniable awakening to the fact that she was in perimenopause. Although changes were evolving for some time, as with most women, they began subtly, often unnoticeably. As knowledgeable as Tara was about the medical field, she had been in denial about her changing menstrual patterns and her changing moods. Different women experience different aspects of their menstrual changes as the eye-opening event of their recognition that something big is happening.

Changes in the menstrual cycle may be the most obvious initial difference in the woman entering perimenopause but there are many other physical changes that accompany or are the result of the changing hormones of perimenopause. The changes in the menstrual cycle are a result of the changing function of the ovaries, which in turn alter the levels of the female hormones in the body. As these changes take hold, the effect becomes global in a woman's system, affecting most systems from the physical to the psychological. Not all women feel or notice these changes; some notice a few changes, some women are affected by many.

Vasomotor Events

Most women (and even most men) are acquainted with the infamous hot flash. The hot flash has historically been believed to be a result of low estrogen levels and rising FSH. Currently, the mechanism believed to create the hot flash is a result of falling estrogen levels but in a far more complex interaction than was previously thought.[28]

The anatomy of the hot flash is vasodilation, or a widening of the blood vessels in the skin that allow for a greater blood flow to the skin of the chest, head and neck. This additional blood flow creates actual heat along with an internal sensation of extreme warmth, often accompanied by sweating that can be profuse. Hot flashes, which affect 75 to 85 percent of women, are frequently followed by chills and typically last approximately four minutes.[29] A hot flash differs from simply feeling overheated on a hot day. The subjective experience of a hot flash is that heat is building up *inside* the body and radiating out. This is a very different sensation than when standing in a warm room or in the sun while heat is bearing down externally. When a woman has a hot flash, the heat becomes trapped in between her skin and her clothing, creating that urgent need to open or remove clothing to allow the heat to escape.

Hot flashes may vary in terms of severity, frequency and duration and are exacerbated by stress.[30] Some women may have a few hot flashes over the course of a week while others report more than ten a day. Hot flash triggers include stress, spicy foods, alcohol, ambient heat, confined spaces, smoking and caffeine. Temperature of the foods and beverages can have an effect on hot flash frequency, as well. In current research women reported suffering more from hot flashes when eating hot foods and drinking hot beverages.[31]

Race is another factor in how one suffers from hot flashes: African American women suffer more while Asian women suffer less.[32] Fortunately, hot flashes are at their most severe for only a few months in most women and resolve completely in 85 to 90 percent of women within five years. Only 10 to 15 percent of women continue to experience hot flashes years after the completion of menopause.[33]

The sister to the hot flash is the night sweat. Caused by the same mechanism as in the hot flash, the night sweat, appropriately named, happens during the night when we are asleep, typically in the early morning hours of 3 to 4 A.M. Night sweats can range from annoying to extremely disruptive. The classic night sweat is like a bad hot flash, causing significant perspiration. They become destructive when they begin to cause frequent, regular disruptions in sleep. This may not only affect a perimenopausal woman, but her bed partner, as well. Most women sleep through many of their night sweats. This was the situation with Jennifer and her husband, Dennis. While Jennifer tossed and turned from four to five sweats each night, Dennis was in an exhausted stupor every day. These women may awaken quite surprised to find their nightclothes on the floor next to the bed or their pajamas on inside out or backwards with no recollection of how this happened!

Both types of vasomotor symptoms, the hot flashes and the night sweats are enormous contributors to both depression and anxiety. Women who have significant vasomotor symptoms have been found to have a six-fold increase in the risk of developing depression.[34] During a vasomotor event, there is also an increase in heart rate, skin temperature and metabolic rate.[35] This can readily set in motion a wave of anxiety.[36] The uninformed woman may simply interpret the physiological changes as anxiety, not understanding they are a result of a vasomotor event.

Often with anxiety, some anxiety begets more anxiety. In simple terms, when an individual feels anxious and does not understand why, they begin to panic as they wonder and fear what is wrong. One woman, Sally, while experiencing frequent hot flashes, would become so anxious, she would experience a claustrophobic sensation. Sally would frantically begin to peel off clothing and run for the nearest exit in order to relieve the panicky feeling.

Night sweats can be managed by turning down the temperature at night and layering clothing and bedding for easy removal. Once the night sweat passes, often women become chilled as the perspiration evaporates and they need to replace pajamas and blankets for warmth. At a recent gathering of couples in which all of the women were in perimenopause, I heard the hilarious complaints of the husbands and their methods of coping with their wive's night sweats. One husband wore a hat and hooded sweatshirt to bed. Another had to wear insulated long underwear used by winter sportsmen, in order to keep warm in the frigid bedrooms their wives needed in the effort to stay cool at night!

Insomnia

Insomnia and sleeplessness are a huge problem in perimenopause, not just due to night sweats but also due to the transition in sleep patterns that come with such a large hormonal shift. Perimenopause-related anxiety is another cause for sleep disruption. What surprises many women is that during the perimenopausal transition, they need an increased amount of sleep, similar to the sleep needs of adolescence. This can contribute to a greater sleep deficit when combined with the sleep loss and sleep disruption in this stage of life. The increased need for sleep will reverse once menopause is complete. While it is present, however, it is very important to try and satisfy what your body needs, even if this means grabbing a nap during the day.

Urogenital Changes

Another major arena for change during perimenopause is in the urogenital arena. The decrease in estrogen causes a thinning of the lining of the urethra and the vagina. This contributes to a reduction in blood supply and a loss of muscle tone to these areas. In the urinary tract this may cause an increase in urinary tract infections and/or urine leakage.[37] It is helpful to wear a panty liner to prevent embarrassment due to leakage when laughing or sneezing or when there is a strong urge to urinate. Rather than eliminating laughter from your life, practicing an exercise, called a Kegel, which involves the tightening and relaxing of vaginal muscles, will help to alleviate this stress incontinence.

The thinning of the lining in the vagina, along with decreased lubrication from the lower levels of estrogen also result in irritation, itching and loss of elasticity in the vaginal tissues. Intercourse may become uncomfortable or even painful. Supplemental lubrication will make sexual encounters more successful.

Table 4-1

Physiological Symptoms of Perimenopause

Menstrual Symptoms
- Erratic Changes in Female Hormones
- Irregular Menstrual Cycles
- Changes in Menstrual Flow
- Breast Tenderness
- Menstrual Migraines

Vasomotor Symptoms
- Hot Flashes
- Night Sweats

Urogenital Symptoms
- Painful Intercourse
- Decrease in Lubrication in Urogenital Tissue
- Itching and Irritation in Vaginal Tissues
- Urinary Tract Infections
- Incontinence

Skin
- Decreased Elasticity in Skin
- Increase in Age Spots

continued...

> *...continued*
> - Increasing in Skin Wrinkles
> - Dryness and Itching in Skin
> - Increase in Skin Sagging
> - Rosacea
>
> **Gastrointestinal**
> - Slowing of Digestion
> - Increase in Intestinal Gas and Bloating
> - Reduction in Saliva Production
>
> **Other**
> - Palpitations
> - Decreasing Bone Density
> - Increased Risk of Cardiovascular Disease
> - Sleep Disturbances
> - Fatigue
> - Insomnia
> - Joint Aches

Skin Changes

During these midlife years, as hormone levels decline, women begin to notice changes in their skin, frequently in the area of skin elasticity.[38] One of the things that upset Carly the most as she went through perimenopause was the loss of her beautiful "porcelain" complexion. No matter what products she tried, her skin was constantly dry and dull. In perimenopause as the skin's production of collagen and elastin decrease, skin becomes less radiant and firm. It will often take on a looser appearance[39] so that lines and creases begin to appear.

Dryness also becomes more of a problem as the oil glands slow down their production. If a woman was a smoker or sun worshipper, this is when the damaging effects begin to show themselves the most.

Another assault on the perimenopausal complexion is the appearance of rosacea. This is a common problem for women during this phase of life. Rosacea is a skin condition of the face and chest, characterized by redness, bumps and small pustules. Rosacea tends to worsen under periods of psychological stress, during the menstrual cycle and will flare in the presence of hot flashes.

If Those Are Not Enough...

There are a number of other physical symptoms associated with perimenopause, easily referenced in Table 4-1. Among them are gastrointestinal problems, such as bloating and gas. Menstrual migraines are frequently a problem right before menstruation, a result of the decline in both estrogen and progesterone before one's period.[40] The breasts become tender and swollen as estrogen levels decline. This is especially true when a woman's progesterone levels have dropped even more than the estrogen levels, a state called "estrogen dominance." During late perimenopause there is an increased rate of reduction in bone density, especially spinal density, causing an increased rate of falling and fractures.[41] Palpitations and increased risk of cardiovascular disease are other problems to watch out for in perimenopause.

Not all of these symptoms show up in every woman. There are women who are plagued by quite a number of these symptoms while others barely notice any changes at all. Data indicates that 20 percent of women suffer no symptoms of perimenopause while another 20 percent suffer severe symptoms.[42] The women, who seem to suffer the most emotionally, are often those who are unaware of what the normal changes in their bodies are and those who are under constant, unrelenting stress. The latter group of women end up in a cycle of physical challenges augmenting emotional challenges, which in turn worsen the physical symptoms, and so on. Fatigue, so characteristic of this stage of life, becomes an additional challenge that makes it infinitely more difficult to manage the stress.

It is critical that women become knowledgeable about what is happening to their bodies and their emotions in order to understand what is normal. Some women find it difficult to handle the aging of their bodies, which appears to speed up during perimenopause. The changes described above, may appear to be a warning that a woman is leaving youth behind and entering "old age." This, too, can become a risk factor for psychological difficulties. Different women opt for different coping strategies. Some will attempt to change their bodies; some will attempt to work on their perspective. Carly considered plastic surgery to improve the appearance of her skin. Her friend had wonderful results doing so. Ultimately, she chose to live with the changes and accept her "new look." A novel perspective that we will learn later is that we exit menopause not as "old" but as reinvented. What is ultimately important, is that every woman passes through this transition with as much knowledge and comfort as she can achieve.

Chapter Five

Am I Becoming a Man?

Many people do not realize that women, not just men, produce androgens, one of which is testosterone. The dominant sex hormones in women, of course, are the estrogens and progesterone. When the changes of perimenopause begin, the ratio of the androgens to estrogen and oxytocin begins to shift, even though there is a net reduction in the amount of androgens. This results in a higher androgen to estrogen ratio with some of the expected results as we see the influence of "male" hormones in our bodies.[43]

Testosterone, in women, as in men, has a significant impact on hair growth. As the perimenopausal shifts in these hormones evolve, women begin to find hair growth patterns on their bodies that can be similar to men. Facial hair may begin to sprout on the upper lip and chin. The fine facial hair that women have prior to these changes may darken and become coarser.

Eleanor, a lovely perimenopausal woman, lamented that every day she must tweeze a half dozen hairs from her chin! Some women find hair growth on their toes and thicker growth on their arms, legs and pubertal area. Simultaneously, many women find their scalp hair thinning, becoming finer and in more extreme cases, mimicking the patterns of male pattern baldness. Naturally, these changes can be very upsetting. Excess hair growth is easily remedied but it is very distressing to women when they suffer significant hair loss.

Increased androgen ratios may also contribute to problems with acne. The erratic hormonal shifts coupled with the emotional stress of perimenopause can create a propensity to developing acne much in the same way as in puberty. Acne, in fact, can be a reliable indicator of the level of androgens in the body.

As we learned in Chapter 3, aggressive behavior is another indicator of the influence of testosterone. Brizendine teaches us that aggression is associated with androgens not just in men, but also in women. For example, the most aggressive teenage females have been shown to have the highest levels of some of the androgens. Within the menstrual cycle, the shifting emotions of social interest, empathy, and desire to connect with others, versus aggression and hostility, change with the lowering and rising androgen levels, respectively.[44]

It becomes easy to deduce that as the balance of testosterone to estrogen begins to shift in favor of testosterone in middle age, the aggressive impulses characteristic of testosterone can become more dominant. As estrogen and oxytocin decline further in later perimenopause, testosterone begins to take on an even more influential role in a woman's emotions. This may be expressed in uncontrolled outbursts of temper, less patience or even sarcasm and irritation. Not only may she be shorter tempered and more easily brought to anger but she will be less likely to be passive in situations that she overlooked earlier in life. These women are more likely to pursue their own agendas, even if it means stepping on some toes.

Simultaneous to the changing ratios of testosterone and estrogen, the reduction in progesterone leaves women without the calming component to the hormone mix, further exposing them to feeling easily agitated and less inclined to nurture.[45] Anyone familiar with a perimenopausal woman has experienced such behavior; virtually every perimenopausal woman is familiar with such feelings.

While the ratio of estrogen to testosterone decreases during perimenopause, as we have learned, the overall amount of testosterone decreases. This creates other complications for the perimenopausal women who may suffer depression as a result of declining testosterone. Some recent research has pointed to declining testosterone more than declining estrogen as a contributor to depression.[46]

The last function of testosterone, we will learn about, is to drive libido. Higher androgen levels increase the sex drive (this is a factor in early teenage promiscuous behavior). Throughout perimenopause testosterone levels decrease by as much as 15 percent.[47] The most significant drops are in the mid-30s and again in the early years of menopause. With this decrease in testosterone, libido can be radically diminished. Between the ages of twenty and menopause, women see a decrease of 60 percent in their testosterone levels. This reduction of testosterone will cause 50 percent of women between the ages of forty-two and fifty-two to actually lose their sex drive.[48] Many women (and their partners) do not understand that this loss of libido is a function of these hormonal changes and instead attribute it to other possibilities, such as loss of interest in their partner.

Chapter Six

When Our "Feel Good" Hormone Fades

*A*s described earlier, progesterone depletion is a major cause of many difficulties in perimenopause. As estrogen levels decline and the LH surge fails to take place, there are an anovulatory cycles that ultimately fail to release progesterone.

Why is progesterone so important?

Progesterone receptors are present throughout the entire body; and its effects are present in every location in which there is a receptor. Because of this, it has global effects in the body. For example, progesterone is a factor in the production of other hormones, including estrogen, testosterone and cortisol. It helps maintain normal thyroid function, promotes healthy bone density, utilizes body fat for fuel and is indicated in the prevention of breast, ovarian and uterine cancers. Progesterone also helps stabilize blood sugar levels, fights heart disease by maintaining proper blood clotting, increases sex drive and of course is a major player in procreation.

One of the more important functions of progesterone is that it counteracts many of the unpleasant effects of estrogen.

We saw earlier how perimenopausal women tend to have fluctuating menstrual flow with an increased frequency of experiencing very heavy menses. This is a result of the decreased progesterone levels. Because progesterone is responsible for regulating the growth of the endometrium in the uterus, when the progesterone levels are low, the endometrium, or uterine lining becomes thicker, resulting in a heavier menstrual flow.

This same process is involved in the development of fibroids in the uterine wall. This is a much more common occurrence in the perimenopausal woman than at any other time of her life. As important as progesterone is, it is not a solo player. As I will explain shortly, this all works in conjunction with the levels of estrogen that become unbalanced in relation to the levels of progesterone. It is believed, though not yet proven, that many of the unpleasant symptoms of perimenopause come from the highly vacillating levels of estrogen in conjunction with the lower levels of progesterone.[49]

In the emotional realm, progesterone plays a very significant role. Progesterone is often referred to as the "feel good hormone." This is because progesterone stabilizes emotions, acting as a natural antidepressant and anxiolytic. It also balances the proliferation of estrogen (which can cause anxiety). Have you ever wondered why women in the late stages of pregnancy report feeling wonderful in spite of the physical discomfort they experience? This is due to the high levels of progesterone. Similarly, progesterone is implicated in postpartum depression as its level drops off dramatically after giving birth.

Cheryl's Hormones

Cheryl decided to become a mother later in life. At the age of 37 she had her first child. Cheryl was happily married to the love of her life. She had spent her twenties as a single woman enjoying life. When she decided to marry and start a family she felt she was ready. Cheryl continued to work after having her first child and was so fulfilled with motherhood, and her life, she and her husband decided to have another child. Sadly, early in her second pregnancy she suffered a miscarriage. Cheryl became very depressed and found it hard to regain her former zest for life. She attributed these feelings completely to the loss of the baby, never considering there may have been a large hormonal component.

Soon enough Cheryl became pregnant again and had a wonderful pregnancy. Her son was born a healthy, calm, sweet baby. Now in her early forties, Cheryl fell into another depression. She could not understand why, when all of her dreams had been fulfilled, and her prayers answered, she felt so unhappy. She began to feel resentful towards her husband and her children and wondered if she had made the wrong choice in starting a family; maybe she was not cut out for motherhood. The resentment, in turn, brought an onslaught of guilt. Cheryl's self-esteem began to plummet as she found it more and more difficult to manage her job, children, household, marriage and most of all, her feelings.

It became obvious that Cheryl was dealing with a complex mix of psychological and physiological problems. She had unresolved emotions surrounding the loss of her pregnancy. She had guilt over splitting her time between her job and her children. She was also having a postpartum depression due to the progesterone drop after the birth of her son. When a year passed and Cheryl still was not herself, I suggested she have hormonal testing. Her periods were still fairly regular but showing the beginning inconsistencies that come with perimenopause. Blood tests revealed that Cheryl was already in perimenopause. Knowing this allowed Cheryl to understand how her physiology was affecting her emotional state. After consulting her doctor she began using progesterone cream to supplement the deficiency in her body. This in conjunction with antidepressants and therapy helped Cheryl to find her way back to enjoying her life.

The effects of progesterone on a woman's mood cannot be underestimated. One again, we can look at the menstrual cycle to have a very clear understanding of how hormones affect how we feel. Upon ovulation, high levels of progesterone are secreted. The sedating effects of progesterone make us feel mellow, impenetrable to stress and even a bit laid back. These are the antidepressant and anxiolytic effects of progesterone, mentioned earlier. Progesterone levels drop off precipitously right before menstruation begins. This is the time in the menstrual cycle that women feel most irritable, temperamental, hostile, depressed, tearful—you name it. Just about any sentimental, intense emotion can be seen at this juncture in the cycle.

When we extrapolate these monthly changes to those in perimenopause, we can begin to understand the psychological and emotional events that women experience. Our bodies are undergoing a long-term, month-by-month withdrawal of progesterone that accelerates over a period of several years. Without the calming effects of progesterone in our systems, at least to the degree we had previously, we become similar to the person who existed in the days prior to menses, but on a daily basis. This barely recognizable woman may be critical, where she used to be tolerant. She may be easily agitated, where typically calm; highly emotional where previously she was unflappable. Not only is she a stranger to her loved ones; she is a stranger to herself.

It is not uncommon for women to suffer serious bouts of anxiety as their bodies suffer the loss of progesterone. Some women experience severe anxiety in circumstances that have never caused them any sort of distress before. One perimenopausal woman, Christine, was confounded by her experience on vacation. She had always been an avid traveler, enjoying many trips to exotic destinations with her husband. As if out of nowhere, she suffered a series of severe panic attacks while on a vacation to a tropical island with her husband. Her anxiety was so severe, she could not enjoy the vacation and only wished to return to the comfort and safety of her home.

For many women in their forties and even late thirties, the hormonal factor is often overlooked when they encounter emotional difficulties. Both Cheryl and Christine are examples of how both the emotional and physiological challenges worked synergistically to create a very difficult situation.

Chapter Seven

Losing our Estrogen, Losing Ourselves?

When most people think about perimenopausal changes, they think about changing hormone levels, changes in bodily appearance, even changes in emotions and feelings. Most individuals do not realize how much changing takes place in a woman's brain due to hormonal and other chemical changes, and how this impacts many of the other changes that unfold in perimenopause.

In the early stages of perimenopause, estrogen levels are vacillating widely. This continues until later in perimenopause when estrogen levels begin to decline. Not only is the body responding to these changing hormone levels, but the brain is, as well. While the brain is exposed to the falling levels of estrogen, in perimenopause the brain also becomes less sensitive to the effects of the estrogen. These shifts in brain chemistry result in differences in the brain's structure and functioning. This, in turn, causes changes throughout the body that bring about emotional and psychological transformations.

Estrogen Makes Us Female

Estrogen is the female hormone that initially triggers the development of the feminine body at puberty. It stimulates the growth of the breast tissues, increases body fat and triggers the growth of the uterine lining that brings about menstruation. Throughout the menstrual cycle in women of all ages, estrogen is responsible for a multitude of symptoms, from physiological to psychological. Changing estrogen levels are responsible for causing headaches, water retention, and upsetting the balance of blood sugar. It is also implicated in raising the risks of both uterine and breast cancer.[50] It promotes clotting of the blood and diminishes the sex drive. Estrogen, when fluctuating, is also instrumental in increasing depression and anxiety.

Our Brains on Estrogen

During puberty the young woman's brain circuitry, fueled by estrogen begins to rewire in significant ways that change the way she thinks, feels and behaves.[51, 52] Estrogen evokes nurturing behavior and motivates the desire to create social networks. It is also the initiator in a young woman's interest in flirting and sexual behavior. The pubescent girl's brain, due to the increase in estrogen, is much more sensitive and responsive to stress especially when it involves relationship issues. This, in turn motivates an avoidance of conflict. All of this can be observed in the unique physiology of the female brain.

Whereas the male brain shows a positive reaction to interpersonal conflict and competition, the female brain shows a negative alert response. These changes, both in the circuitry of the brain and the emotional behavior of the individual, are all a result of the influx of estrogen.[53]

Another role estrogen has is in affecting the cyclic variations in cognition and mood.[54] It has "neuroprotective effects,"[55] hence, is responsible for stabilizing fluctuating moods. In one study, women in early perimenopause, a time of widely fluctuating estrogen levels, showed a statistically significant increase in mood variability, including nervousness, irritability and in some women, dysphoric mood compared to premenopausal women.[56] The effect of vacillating estrogen on mood is worsened as progesterone declines because of progesterone's moderating effects on estrogen.

Since estrogen is a major factor in the biochemical functioning of the brain as well as the structure of the brain, decreasing estrogen exerts its effects in these areas, as well.[57] The 'psychoendocrine theory' describes how exposure to different sex hormones in the intrauterine environment creates different circuitry and brain structures for the different sexes. This in turn creates different cognitive abilities in males and females.

What are women's strengths? Verbal skills and memory, fine motor abilities, perceptual speed and accuracy are some of the areas in which women outperform men. Men tend to excel on tasks that involve visual memory, mathematical and spatial tasks.[58] When the young boy or girl reaches puberty, the onslaught of sex hormones activates the neural circuitry laid down prenatally. These sex hormones continue their activational effects as long as those hormones circulate in the body.[59]

Going Backwards?

As the estrogen levels in the body decrease throughout perimenopause, the brain's structure and function, once again, begin to shift. One of the cognitive abilities that is compromised, as expected, is verbal memory[60, 61] and learning.[62] How frequently do perimenopausal women find themselves searching their memories for that word or name that they just cannot seem to bring into focus? Women who previously prided themselves on their recall find this new challenge very disconcerting.

Take the embarrassing story of Amy. Amy was on a rant searching the house for her keys…only to find them in the refrigerator, comfortably nestled in between the cheese and the soy!

Amanda, a forty-seven year old patient of mine, was so distraught and frustrated with the shift in her cognition and recall, she was convinced she was developing Alzheimer's Disease. Denise, another woman in her late forties, was sure she had Attention Deficit Disorder. Both of these women remained unconvinced that these symptoms were a result of changing hormone levels with the subsequent changes in the brain's structure. Both women insisted on neurological and psychological testing before they were convinced.

When women begin to notice and experience such changes, especially in the absence of an understanding that this is a normal part of the changes of perimenopause, they will be vulnerable to experiencing an increase in anxiety. This complicates the situation even further, since high levels of anxiety are known to interfere with cognitive performance and memory.[63] The anxiety worsens the symptoms with which one is already struggling. Understanding and accepting these natural changes can help mitigate the frustrations they present. This becomes a time to invoke new strategies for supporting one's sluggish memory. In our modern society, all sorts of electronic devices are available for this effort. For the technologically challenged, we still have the old fashioned, overstuffed, scribbled in appointment book!

Two other hormones that decline along with estrogen are oxytocin and testosterone. Oxytocin, similar to estradiol, a hormone that induces nurturing, calming, and quieting, both in feeling and in behavior is reduced. This leaves women feeling less maternal and less patient in ways that are often foreign to them and their loved ones. It also leaves women without the protection against stressors that they previously had with high oxytocin levels. The good news is that oxytocin is released when women are stroked or massaged. Interestingly, oxytocin will be released when a woman pets a dog, not just in her, but oxytocin will be released in the dog, as well!

We have already learned that a reduction in testosterone levels can radically diminish a woman's sex drive. The reduction in estrogen, oxytocin and testosterone together, spells trouble for a woman's emotional state, degree of reactivity, perception of reality, and ability to cope, in general. No wonder women subjected to these changes are much more prone towards depression and anxiety!

Hot Flashes and Heart Health

What other havoc does diminishing estrogen wreak on our bodies? One of the most talked about challenges of declining estrogen is the notorious "hot flash." Hot flashes are present in 79 percent of perimenopausal women,[64] and yes, they do occasionally follow you into the postmenopausal years. The physiology of the hot flash is a skin temperature increase of four to eight degrees coinciding with an increase in internal body temperature. Hot flashes can be bothersome during the daytime or nighttime hours. A woman having a hot flash has a feeling of warmth that may be subtle or extreme. She may perspire lightly or sweat like an athlete. In most cases, they are unpleasant, at best.

Julia, while going through a period of frequent hot flashes, had no sympathy for her husband who complained that when she touched him, she felt burning hot. This was a result of a measurable change in her external body temperature.

Interestingly, there are a number of factors that contribute to the severity of hot flashes. Weight is one of them. Heavier women may suffer more from the symptoms of a hot flash because the extra subcutaneous fat interferes with the dissipation of heat. Conversely, some research indicates that women who are thin have trouble with hot flashes because they have fewer fat cells that make and store estrogen.[65] This excess estrogen can be utilized during perimenopause, when the ovaries are making less estrogen. Hence, the fat cells counteract some of the effects of estrogen loss in perimenopause. The thin woman has fewer fat cells with less estrogen reserve and therefore suffers more severe symptoms of estrogen depletion. Maybe those extra pounds we seem to gain in perimenopause will be put to good use!

Night sweats, or nocturnal hot flashes are extremely disruptive to sleep,[66] bringing us to another very common complaint of the perimenopausal woman, that of exhaustion. Decreased estrogen levels disrupt REM sleep , the last stage of sleep in which dreaming occurs. While we are losing sleep due to the effects of night sweats, we are also experiencing sleep disruptions from changes in our sleep cycle. We will learn more about the intricate interactions of disrupted sleep and a host of peri-menopausal symptoms in Chapter 9.

As estrogen levels begin to decline with the onset of perimenopause, many of the benefits of higher estrogen levels begin to decline, as well. One of these lost benefits is that the risk for heart disease increases. Lower estrogen levels actually tend to increase low-density lipoprotein (LDL) cholesterol, the "bad" cholesterol and decrease high-density lipoprotein (HDL) cholesterol, the "good" cholesterol. Both of these changes increase the risk for developing heart disease.[67] Along with the increased risk of heart disease, declining estrogen levels increase the risk of developing osteopenia or osteoporosis as it contributes to a reduction in bone density. This can be a great reason to start that exercise and healthy eating program you have been putting off. Your body needs special attention now, more than ever before, to ensure that your entry into the postmenopausal years is a healthy one.

Chapter Eight

First Alert:
When Estrogen Takes Over

Estrogen dominance is one of the more troublesome aspects of perimenopause. When the progesterone levels are low due to the absence of the developed corpus luteum, as explained earlier, estrogen is present unopposed or unbalanced by progesterone. This condition of estrogen dominance can be present whether estrogen levels have or have not fallen from their normal levels prior to perimenopause. This is because the ratio of the estrogen to progesterone is what is important, not simply the amounts. The woman's body behaves as if there is a surplus of estrogen because it is not appropriately balanced by progesterone. Estrogen excesses may also be experienced when the ovaries attempt to "discard" the remaining eggs by attempting to ripen several follicles in a cycle. This is the body's mechanism to protect against old eggs becoming fertilized. Perimenopause brings about the disposal of the store of eggs. Again, these eggs are not likely to fully mature, the ovulation process is incomplete and there will be no production of progesterone.[68]

Estrogen dominance creates symptoms that will alert a woman to the changes happening in her body (see Table 8-1). It is commonly the cause of the irregularity in the woman's menstrual cycle and frequently causes excessive bleeding during menstruation. This can take the form of increased menstrual flow (remember Tara from Chapter 4 who suffered from flooding) or an elongated duration of flow. Often a woman will experience both. It is not uncommon for a woman to have a period lasting two weeks when estrogen is dominant in perimenopause.

Patricia's Periods

Patricia knew she had begun perimenopause. Her periods had been atypical for some time. She had begun to notice differences in the way she felt, in general, but specifically her periods were becoming less and less regular. Patricia had always had very heavy periods. She knew her own pattern: first day, not too heavy, moderate cramping. Her second day was her worst: very heavy flow with some very uncomfortable cramping. From the third day through the seventh, the flow gradually eased into a light spotting with no further discomfort.

Increasingly, Patricia noticed the pattern shifting. Instead of the thirty-two day cycle she had had since age thirteen, Patricia began menstruating anywhere from twenty-eight to thirty-nine days apart. Sometimes her period lasted a week, but more often it lasted nine, ten, up to fourteen days. She noticed she now had to double her protection, wearing a sanitary napkin and tampon on her heaviest days. Patricia was fortunate in having a circle of friends who were open about perimenopausal changes. They shared stories and reading materials. Although these menstruation changes did not come as a surprise to Patricia, they were still quite troublesome and disconcerting. Having her period at times up to three weeks out of four was simply not fun!

When women are experiencing estrogen dominance, the premenstrual days are often much more uncomfortable than at any prior time. All of the 'typical' symptoms of PMS (premenstrual syndrome) may be compounded and much more extreme. Women who have never suffered from PMS find that for the first time they do. They may experience bloating with excess weight gain along with swelling and soreness in their breasts. They will be vulnerable to mood swings, irritability and depressive symptoms before they begin menstruating. Painful abdominal cramping is also common in the estrogen dominant woman. In addition to these uncomfortable symptoms, many women develop premenstrual headaches that are sometimes quite severe. It is not uncommon for women to develop migraines, occasionally for several days on end.

Another common complaint of women who have estrogen dominance is the difficulty losing weight and developing fat on their abdomens, hips and thighs. Their preferred method of weight loss no longer works as effectively. Their tried and true exercise routine produces inadequate results. If this is not difficult enough an increase in sugar and chocolate cravings are an added challenge. This comes at a time when the body is most likely to have difficulty processing sugar, carbohydrates and caffeine.

Yet another troublesome feature of the abundance of estrogen relative to progesterone is that there is frequently a noticeable dampening effect on a woman's sex drive. As we have already learned, declining levels of androgens (one of which is testosterone) compound this effect. Many women feel a significantly reduced urge to have sexual relations while some lose their sex drive completely.[69] Alternatively, many women report an increased desire for cuddling and other forms of physical affection. As we learned in the prior chapter, oxytocin is released during stroking and cuddling. This has a calming effect on a woman, very much needed when she is estrogen dominant.

Women need to be aware of two common medical issues that may develop as a result of estrogen dominance. The first is the development of uterine fibroids, the second is a higher incidence of fibroids in the breasts (also called fibroadenomas or fibrocystic breast disease). Finding fibroids can create a very stressful situation especially when it may require invasive testing or surgical removal. Uterine fibroids may require removal if they become too large or contribute to excessive bleeding. Occasionally, fibroids in the breast that look suspicious may require a biopsy. More typically these fibroids are not a cause for concern. When menopause is complete and the estrogen levels decline dramatically, the fibroids usually shrink and may even disappear. These challenges of perimenopause become contributors to the anxiety and depression to which the perimenopausal woman is already susceptible.

Table 8-1
Symptoms of Estrogen Dominance[70]

- Irregular Menstrual Periods
- Water Retention
- Breast Swelling and tenderness
- Worsening of PMS Symptoms
- Decrease in Sex Drive
- Mood Swings (Depression, Anxiety, Irritability)
- Hastening of Aging
- Thinning Hair
- Weight Gain
- Increase in Fat Deposits (especially on stomach, hips and thighs)
- Increased Risk of Breast Cancer
- Increased Risk of Fibroids or Cysts in Breasts, Ovaries and Uterus
- Increased Risk of Uterine Cancer
- Headaches and Migraines

continued...

...continued

- Slowed Metabolism
- Exhaustion
- Insomnia
- Sluggish Memory
- Blood Sugar Irregularities
- Risk of Thyroid Irregularities
- Reduction in Immune Function

Chapter Nine

Sleep Is Not Just Sleeping:
Sleep Challenges and Dreaming

An extremely common complaint of women in perimenopause is that of disrupted sleep. It is so common in the over forty woman that it is a nearly universal complaint. Not all women suffer from chronic sleep disruptions, but many suffer from occasional disruptions. Research indicates as many as 77 percent of perimenopausal women experience insomnia[71] while only one third of them believe that their sleep difficulties are related to menopause.[72] Disrupted sleep is enough of a problem at any time, but perimenopause is a time of life when most women need additional sleep.

Experts stand by the belief that the typical person needs a full eight hours of sleep per night.[73, 74] The United States is a sleep deprived nation. People average less than seven hours with one third of people getting less than six and a half hours.[75] When considering the forty-plus woman, who now needs more than eight hours of sleep, sometimes as much as nine or ten hours, and how little she is getting, the problem becomes obvious. At this juncture, the forty plus, perimenopausal woman, is not unlike the adolescent. Just as the adolescent's increased need for sleep must be satisfied, so must this woman's. Her increasing sleep debt cannot be ignored without suffering uncomfortable, even dangerous consequences.

Insomnia manifests in three primary ways: *initial insomnia*, when an individual has trouble falling asleep, *middle insomnia*, characterized by awakening in the middle of the night, one or more times, combined with having trouble returning to sleep and finally, *terminal insomnia*, when one awakens too early and cannot return to sleep at all. Even when acquiring a sufficient number of hours of sleep, a woman suffering from one of the disrupted sleep patterns may awaken feeling exhausted, fatigued and not at all refreshed.

Sleep disruptions are caused by and interwoven with many of the other events that occur at this perimenopausal/midlife juncture. Some of these include thyroid problems, which will be discussed in detail in Part III, vasomotor events (hot flashes and night sweats), frequent urination, emotional issues such as anxiety and depression, general life issues and prolific and intense dreaming. Understanding these issues, how they influence one another and how to manage them will be discussed in this chapter.

Vasomotor Events:
How Can I Sleep in a Steam Room?

Much attention has been given to the role vasomotor events play in increasing insomnia.[76, 77] Vasomotor symptoms are more commonly called "flushes", "hot flashes" and "night sweats." They result from falling estrogen levels and the reduction in progesterone production that is characteristic of perimenopause.

When a woman has a vasomotor event, she will perspire, her heart and metabolic rates will increase, along with an increase in the temperature of her skin and her internal core.[78] Nocturnal hot flashes, or "night sweats," can produce extreme amounts of perspiration and sweating and are highly linked to perimenopausal insomnia because of the extreme discomfort they induce. Some research indicates that vasomotor events tend to trigger middle insomnia the most.[79] Chronic insomnia, insomnia lasting at least six months, has been highly correlated with hot flashes; affecting 80 percent of women who suffer from severe hot flashes, even those as young as thirty-five.[80] Changes in overall sleep stage patterns are also associated with night sweats, resulting in general sleep disruption and reduced sleep efficiency.[81] It is easy to see why women awaken exhausted and fatigued.

Women suffering from hot flashes often find it difficult to distinguish whether the heat they are experiencing is internally or externally produced; hence the all too familiar question, "Is it hot in here, or is it me?" When the hot flash presents as a night sweat, women awaken feeling as if they have been placed in a steam room. This incredibly uncomfortable phenomenon can leave a woman feeling extremely hot with mild to copious amounts of sweating. Awakening to find her hair, sheets or pajamas soaking wet is not uncommon.

By using a combination of self-report questionnaires and external monitoring equipment, one very interesting study found that women sleep through about half of their nighttime hot flashes.[82] In other words, women were not even aware of 50 percent of their night sweats. This may explain the phenomenon experienced by Dana. Dana, who enjoyed sleeping in her comfortable pajama bottoms and T-shirt, awoke one morning to find her T-shirt on inside out and backwards. She was certainly amused to realize that during her nightly sweats, and subsequent chills she had taken off her bedclothes and dressed herself again without ever awakening!

Other women have awakened to find blankets removed and evidently replaced in a manner indicating interesting happenings during the night. Happily, women are blessed with not having to suffer from full awakenings with every night sweat. Sadly, however, women do suffer the effects of such turbulent nights with sleepiness and even exhaustion the following day.

So, What Can I Do?

Many women find some relief by employing a few preventive measures. *Keeping your bedroom as cool as possible* is a good way to start. Remember to tell your frozen spouse that he can easily add a few layers of clothing. There is nothing wrong with going to bed with socks and gloves! If you get better sleep, he will benefit almost as much as you will, maybe even more. In this vein, you can also turn on a fan. The movement of circulating air is often enough to reduce or ward off a hot flash. A ceiling fan over your bed is a wonderful solution.

Utilize layers. Layer everything from blankets to bedclothes. A heavy blanket or outer layer of pajamas can be easily removed as a night sweat sets in. Be sure to keep them close by. When you are finished heating up, you will cool down and want those layers back.

Avoid caffeine altogether if possible, but certainly after lunchtime. Caffeine is a culprit in increasing hot flashes and night sweats. It is also counterproductive for rest and relaxation. Caffeine can be found in the obvious places of coffee and sodas but may also be present in desserts, chocolate, teas or other beverages. When you have difficulty sleeping, caffeine is likely to exacerbate your troubles.

Finally, *calm down!* Anxiety has been known to increase the frequency and severity of vasomotor events.[83] A mild night sweat can degenerate into a full blown 'steam room event' when a woman awakens and becomes anxious from the sensations she is experiencing. This, in turn, can severely disrupt a night of restful sleep as the anxiety worsens the vasomotor event, which in turn increases anxiety further. In this regard, women who are inclined towards nighttime anxiety may benefit from taking a small amount of an anxiolytic medication at bedtime. This can be in the form of a prescription medication, such as a benzodiazepine. It can also be in the form of an over the counter supplement including anything from a cup of warm milk or chamomile tea, to herbal supplements such as valerian root or kava kava. These are helpful alternatives to taking hormones when a woman experiences anxiety that exacerbates night sweats and ruins night after night of restful sleep.

One of the more critical problems issuing from sleep disturbances is the decrease in healthy psychological functioning, especially in perimenopausal women. Both anxiety and depression have been associated with disrupted sleep.[84, 85] Sleep deprivation, even a nominal amount, has been proven to create mood shifts including a higher risk of depression and a lower threshold for anger and irritability.[86] A greater sensitivity to emotional issues and feelings of being unable to cope along with increased anxiety are all common results of sleep deprivation and insomnia.[87] Many perimenopausal women already suffer from excessive worry, anxiety and of having a "shorter fuse." While the hormonal challenges have a strong negative impact on these emotional issues, sleep challenges add another level of disruption to women's sense of wellbeing.

Tired Theresa

Theresa's story typifies this dynamic. Theresa is a single mother of a teenager. Barely forty, she was already noticing changes in her menstrual cycle. Although Theresa worked in the medical field, she was in denial that she was in the beginning stages of perimenopause. What Theresa did admit was that she was perpetually exhausted. A typical night involved several awakenings. When she awakened in the early morning hours, she was frequently unable to return to sleep. Theresa readily acknowledged the presence of stresses from her job and her personal life. She attributed her difficulty sleeping and ever-present fatigue to those stresses.

After nearly a year of regular nighttime difficulties, Theresa's increasing irritability had developed into debilitating anxiety. She felt a knot in her stomach continually, was hypersensitive to any infraction by another and felt as though life was just too difficult to cope with. She had begun to have problems with her coworkers. At her age, how could she afford to be burned out? She was financially responsible for herself and her son and certainly could not be calling it quits at this point.

> *Upon closer examination, Theresa acknowledged she had been having some night sweats. The night sweats were often the cause of her frequent awakenings. The distress this caused, coupled with her general state of anxiety, interfered with her ability to return to sleep. Theresa had entered that vicious cycle of sleep deprivation leading to exhaustion, which created irritability and anxiety that intensified sleep disruption, and so on.*

The converse of this phenomenon is also true. Not only does sleep deprivation make women more susceptible to mood disorders but anxiety and other mood disturbances adversely affect sleep.[88] Terminal insomnia indicates the presence of depression[89] while anxiety often causes initial insomnia. Stress, emotional and mental tension in those suffering from anxiety can be so overwhelming, they hamper or even prevent sleep onset.[90] The many psychosocial difficulties that are present in midlife can create enough distress that they, too, can be potent disruptors of restful sleep.

A very troublesome aspect of this relationship between mood disorders, specifically anxiety, and sleep is when they become interwoven in an escalating manner. When a stressed individual has trouble falling asleep, she may begin to engage in what John Harvey, psychologist and relaxation specialist calls "sleep-ruining thoughts" or SRTs.[91] SRTs are the anxious thoughts that commonly develop once an individual has suffered from some sleep difficulties. The common SRTs are really anxieties that past sleep difficulties will become future difficulties. Examples are:

- "I know I won't be able to fall asleep again tonight," or,
- "If I don't get a good night's sleep tonight, I'll be unable to function tomorrow," or even,
- "I had better not awaken tonight because I won't be able to fall back to sleep."

These anxious thoughts become an integral part of the pattern of escalating sleep problems. In a very stressed individual, it may take only one night of poor sleep to initiate a nightly ritual of bedtime anxiety that becomes a saboteur of restful sleep thereafter. Before long, the anxiety can back up into daytime hours, as well. Starting early in the day, the anxiety levels build as bedtime approaches and the concern over sleeping increases.

How Life Events Impact Sleep

We are beginning to understand how the many significant life events that unfold at this juncture in a woman's life intersect. Hormonal changes, stress and depression all contribute to disrupted sleep patterns,[92] but psychosocial and psychodynamic changes can impinge on healthy sleep, as well. Depending on what age a woman was when she started her family, she may be coping with her children entering puberty just as she enters perimenopause. This leaves her with the challenge of managing her children's rapidly changing hormones, moods and stability at the same time she has to understand and manage her own.

A woman who had children at a younger age may have her children leaving home for college or independent living when she enters this milestone. This will set in motion a domino effect of changing relationships with her husband and friends. Such a situation requires her to recreate her priorities, her sense of purpose and her role with her spouse. All of these impingements have the potential of intruding on her ability to enter into healthy restful sleep. Many of these struggles may find their way into her dreams, as was the case with Margie.

Margie's Dreams

Margie began having a recurring dream in her mid forties. It was not quite a nightmare, but certainly was a very disturbing dream. Typically after having one or another version of this dream, Margie felt unsettled for the better part of the day. The underlying theme of the dream was that of Margie finding herself in school.

Sometimes it was high school, sometimes college. In every version, Margie was attempting to attend classes but had lost her schedule. Each version of the dream offered a different impediment to her finding or acquiring a new schedule. In some cases she could not find the office where she could get a new schedule. In other cases she would face a humiliating or punitive outcome in requesting the replacement schedule.

The pressure Margie felt to get to her classes was enormous and quite disturbing. She knew she had already missed some classes and a lot of work. She knew it would be disastrous to miss more. There was a sense in the dream of impending doom if she did not get this problem resolved quickly. She saw herself wandering the halls, watching all of the other students hurrying towards their appropriate classrooms. Everyone else knew where he or she was supposed to be. Only Margie stood there in a state of helpless confusion, feeling totally obvious, yet invisible at the same time. She was desperate to find where she belonged; yet every avenue to reconciling the problem was blocked in some way. As the dream progressed, Margie felt increasingly lost and distraught.

Margie's dream reflected her true-life feelings of being lost. Margie knew she was perimenopausal. An open person, who spoke freely with her friends, Margie was quite familiar with the changes happening in her body. Her passage through these hormonal shifts seemed to have a greater effect on her than most of her friends reported experiencing. This left her feeling somewhat isolated. She was also struggling with an enormous life change as the last of her children became independent. While she and her husband had a very strong relationship, all of these changes put stress on this part of her life, as well. Nothing was as it should be; nothing was as it had been before.

Her dreams tells us of the powerful motivation she had to sort things out. It also speaks to us of the enormous frustration in doing so. Margie needed to figure out where she belonged. In the dream, the classroom schedule symbolized Margie's changing roles in her life. She continued to dream versions of this dream, each exploring a different angle of the same problem. It was difficult for Margie to suffer through exhausting days following the disrupted sleep of those turbulent nights, but Margie worked in conjunction with the subconscious thrust of her feelings to find a more harmonious place for herself.

In addition to the many challenges presented by growing children and changing partner relationships, another troublesome life event for the forty something woman may be her parents. Adults at this stage of life are referred to as the 'sandwich generation' since they are sandwiched between the needs of their dependent children and their aging parents who are frequently becoming less independent and more dependent. Many women discover there is a role reversal in their relationships with their parents as they may find themselves taking charge and making decisions for their parents as they become sick or elderly. Psychologically, this can be frightening as it is not easy to become your parents' parent. Emotionally, a woman may feel abandoned as she realizes that at this very difficult juncture in her life, her parents may not be able to be there for her.

Sleep and Concentration

Dr. James Maas,[93] a prominent sleep expert, compares the adequacy of sleep to a bank account. If you are sleep deprived, the result is a sleep debt that needs to be repaid. Since most people require eight hours and perform optimally with ten hours of sleep per night, and since few get that much, the majority of adults have a sleep debt that accumulates over time. Living with a sleep dept has a negative impact on functioning. What is this negative impact? Maas lists inattentiveness, an inclination to make mistakes and an increase in accidents as risks of sleep debt. Alternatively, enhanced vigilance, energy, information processing, creativity and critical thinking are increased with optimal sleep.

Now let us examine the perimenopausal woman from this perspective. We already know that sleep is more disrupted and overall sleep quantity and quality is reduced during this stage of life. When we apply the findings of the sleep experts to the behaviors and difficulties of the forty plus woman, we find some interesting explanations for troubling phenomena.

Take Suzie who found the container of orange juice in the cupboard where she keeps her drinking glasses. Sadly for Suzie, there was no one but herself at home, leaving no one but herself to blame. How about Pam, who spent two days looking for the money she received from a charity collection, only to realize she had not actually attended the charity function that particular day. Perhaps the most painful of these lapses in concentration was that of Cindy who ran out of her office to get something to eat. Unfortunately, it was the most expensive meal of her life since Cindy left her keys on her desk. Embarrassment was the least of her problems as she handed a locksmith $250 of her hard-earned income to get her back inside!

These lapses in concentration, vigilance and clear thinking are characteristic of women in this age range. The question is, how many of them are due to hormonal changes and how many are due to sleep disruption and insomnia. As of now, we do not have an answer to that question, but we do know that each makes a significant contribution. The presence of both the hormonal changes and the sleep disruption that interfere with focus and concentration can create a very challenging situation.

Dreaming

Many perimenopausal women not only have trouble falling asleep and maintaining restful sleep, but also report an increased amount of highly detailed, elaborate and emotionally impacting dreams. The "pregnancy dream" is extremely common in the perimenopausal years. Jerilynn Prior, a researcher on women's hormonal changes, attributes this to an increase in estrogen levels during the initial stages of perimenopause.[94]

Mindy's Struggle

Mindy had always been a prolific dreamer, but even that did not prepare her for the intensity of the dreams she began having in perimenopause. Some of the dreams were so penetrating and powerful; they left Mindy feeling out of sorts for the entire day. A common theme in Mindy's dreams was pregnancy.

Early in perimenopause, Mindy was having dreams of being pregnant that were so realistic; she would often awaken momentarily believing she was, in fact, pregnant. An odd sense of feeling connected to a state of pregnancy stayed with her throughout the day and sometimes for several days afterwards. In most of these dreams, Mindy felt comforted by the pregnancies and awakened with a happy, reminiscent feeling for her own real pregnancies. Over time, the happy, contented feeling she had had from these dreams began to shift into an unsettled, wistful longing for the wonderful childbearing years of her life.

Psychologically, Mindy was reprocessing her childbearing years. She was aware on a conscious and unconscious level that her ability to bear children was coming to a close. The dreams represented a connection to a time of her life that was wonderful and fulfilling. Only in her dreams could she comfortably revisit the wonderful feelings associated with pregnancy and bearing children.

As perimenopause progressed, Mindy's dreams took an odd turn. She continued to dream she was pregnant, but rather than giving birth to beautiful babies, she would find herself birthing beautiful puppies and kittens. In her dreams, she would progress through a "typical" pregnancy. When the puppies and kittens were born, she would be excited and thrilled, similar to how she had been when having babies.

This stage in Mindy's passage through perimenopause shows us how, unconsciously, she was moving towards a reconciliation of the termination of her ability to bear children. In giving birth to puppies and kittens, Mindy, an animal lover, was preparing to find substitutes for the ability to fill her life with her own human babies. The animals represent a healthy adaptation to finding a new way to fulfill her maternal needs. She might not be able to have children, but she could still bring other types of "babies" into her life.

Towards the end of Mindy's perimenopause, as she inched closer and closer to menopause, the content of Mindy's pregnancy dreams shifted again. This time, Mindy dreamed she was large and bloated, as if well into pregnancy. She had all of the discomforts of a late stage pregnancy, but knew there was no baby within her. In her dreams, she wished, impatiently, that this uncomfortable state would soon be over. If she could only figure out how to hasten it, she would be happy.

Here we see Mindy's full, unconscious reconciliation of her diminished fertility. Mindy's desire to be done with the uncomfortable state of pseudo-pregnancy tells us that she was ready to accept her completion of perimenopause and the infertility it would bring. No longer was she wishing in her dreams to revisit her former pregnancies. She was now finished, eager and capable of moving on.

Not only is it common for women in perimenopause to dream about pregnancy, but they also frequently dream about menstruating. These dreams may also be disconcerting. Women have reported dreams in which they are getting their period but have no pads or tampons available, where flow may be excessive or they may be in situations that threaten to embarrass them. When there is an element of frustration or anxiety about the dreams that stays with them after awakening, we know there is unconscious work being done.

Women in perimenopause may dream so realistically that they have begun menstruating, that they awaken, running to the bathroom to check. Alternately, women may dream about the absence of their menses.

Some women tell of dreams in which they are waiting interminably for their periods to begin. These dreams, also, tend to have an anxious sense about them. The dream content may contain all sorts of life issues that are impinged upon due to the presence or absence of the menstrual cycle. It is important to keep in mind that perimenopause is a time of enormous physical and psychological change. The managing of this change will undoubtedly find its way into one's dreams.

As straightforward as they may seem, not all dreams are obvious in their meaning. Even dreams that seem to be absolutely obvious, contain a wealth of symbolic content. Dreams that represent the transition from fertility and menstruation to infertility and menopause may appear with all sorts of symbolic content, some that are seemingly unrelated to the issue at hand. For example, one perimenopausal woman, Jody, dreamt that she wanted to have sex with her husband. Every attempt she made to either create the romantic environment or connect with him met with some sort of obstacle. She felt increasingly frustrated and desperate in the dream as she made more unsuccessful attempts to be with him.

The clue that there was important unconscious meaning was the extraordinary distress Jody felt upon awakening and throughout the following day. The distress was disproportionate to the surface content of the dream. In analyzing her dream, Jody realized that as her cycles became irregular, the pattern of her sexual desire became foreign to her. This had a definite and uncomfortable impact on her sexual relationship with her husband. Jody began to feel insecure about her future as a sexual woman, especially about when the time would come that she would cease menstruating entirely. This expanded into concern about the future of her relationship with her husband and the viability of her marriage.

Multiple dreams with varying content may be expressions of the same issue. An important issue may take many nights and many dreams to find expression.[95] As Freud explains, (dreaming) "…makes possible early recognition of bodily changes which in waking life would still for a time have remained unnoticed,"[96] It is only when the dreamer is psychologically ready to acknowledge the meaning of the dream content that she will remember and understand it.

Interesting Sleep Facts

- When women are premenstrual, they sleep less.
- Women have more nightmares than men have.
- Women experiencing night sweats are more likely to have nightmares.
- Women are more susceptible to suffering from insomnia than are men.
- The phase of a woman's menstrual cycle influences the sexual content of her dreams.
- Menopausal women experience less sexual content in their dreams.
- Progesterone has direct anesthetic and hypnotic properties, facilitating restful sleep.[97]
- Many psychological problems in perimenopause are a result of sleep deprivation. [98]

Part II

The Volatile Psychology of Perimenopause and Life in the Forties

In perimenopause the changes of puberty are in a sense reversing. The hormones that began to surge in the pre-adolescent woman are now beginning to diminish. Similar to the rocky up and down spurts of both estrogen and progesterone that mark the transition into puberty, so is there such an irregular pattern of surging and spurting of estrogen and progesterone on the path of their decline. This does not mean that women cease to be feminine but that some of the estrogen induced behaviors do not feel as dominant or as comfortable. The progesterone-induced feelings also begin to change in an irregular pattern leaving a woman with feelings and emotions that are alien to her. It is my hope that as women began to understand how the physiological changes that are happening in their bodies interact with their feelings and emotions, they will be more confident and comfortable as they pass through this very challenging transition in life. I have often observed that it is the lack of knowledge that fuels the fears that so many women experience as they muddle through perimenopause. Once women understand what to expect, what is normal and how they can handle some of what they are experiencing, the psychological difficulties become much more manageable and women cope infinitely better.

As we have already seen, Part I of this book focuses on the physiology of perimenopause. This section, Part II focuses on the psychology of perimenopause. Table 0-2 lists the common psychological symptoms many perimenopausal women experience. I want to reiterate that these two aspects of perimenopause are not mutually exclusive. There are clearly interactional components between the physiological and psychological aspects of perimenopause that are bidirectional, each one influencing the other. The understanding of the process of how the physiological and psychological changes in a perimenopausal individual mutually affect one another is in its infancy. Ongoing research continues to broaden our knowledge about this process. This will be explored in more detail later.

Table 0-2

Psychological Symptoms of Perimenopause

- Despondency
- Nervousness
- Irritability
- Fatigue
- Insomnia
- Forgetfulness
- Low Self-Esteem
- Decreased Libido

continued...

...continued

- Sadness
- Feeling Overwhelmed
- Inertia
- Confusion
- Loss of Identity
- Self-doubt
- Conflict
- Loneliness
- Poor Concentration
- Hopelessness
- Fearfulness
- Worrying
- Panic
- Relationship Problems
- Anger
- Impulsivity
- Distress

Chapter Ten

Psychological Stages
of Perimenopause

I have delineated four psychological stages of perimenopause that reflect the emotional experiences of women in perimenopause. It is important to understand that the psychological changes do not always coincide with the physiological changes, which are subject to great variability. After speaking to and working with many perimenopausal women, I have determined that there is a typical transition, psychologically and emotionally, from beginning to end. Not all women will share the same intensity of feelings and experiences, but most will follow this pattern. Some women will have more difficulty with one stage versus another, while others may experience equal intensity in every stage. There are many women who sail through perimenopause with very little psychological impact. There are women who struggle every step of the way.

In this chapter, I hope to give women some comfort by knowing what to expect in each stage and how they will progress to an endpoint that every woman can anticipate with relief and joy. By breaking down the progression of emotional change into stages from the beginning to the end of perimenopause, it will be easier for women to understand what they are experiencing. The stages also serve to help women assess where they are in the perimenopausal progression.

Stage I: Perimenopausal Initiation

New indications reveal that the earliest onset of perimenopause is sooner than anyone had previously thought. Women in their middle to late thirties may already be experiencing the subtle changes associated with this transition. These women are not remotely thinking about being near perimenopause or menopause. They would probably consider you crazy if you tried to make such a suggestion.

Menstruation

In this stage, women will not notice any changes in their menstrual cycle, nor will they experience hot flashes or night sweats. They may find a slightly increased unpleasantness associated with the premenstrual phase of their cycle. The primary indication of the beginning onset of hormonal change will be in the subtle shift in a woman's mood and degree of patience.

Moods

The women I have treated that are in Stage I, Perimenopausal Initiation, find their threshold for tolerating unpleasantness or distress is slightly lower. Their reactivity is a bit quicker and slightly more intense than ever before. Often, these women will interpret this change as a result of the increased demands in their lives or the disappointments and frustrations they experience from spouses or children. Women will often describe a sense of feeling saturated, that they have had enough of: their husbands not picking up after themselves, not helping with the housework or needing to be told what to do instead of figuring it out for themselves. Mothers will be fed up with having to tell their children to do their homework, clean their rooms or clear the table. She may have fantasies of taking a weekend vacation alone, while someone cooks, cleans and makes her bed so she can shop, relax or read a book, undisturbed. She finds herself slightly less patient than ever before.

As women, we all understand that such frustrations are common in the lives of wives and mothers. The difference between ordinary frustration and the feelings of the women in Perimenopausal Initiation is primarily a matter of intensity and the ability to cope. Before a woman has begun the hormonal changes of perimenopause, she is more inclined to take these stresses in stride. Once in this stage of perimenopause, she will find herself more likely to feel overwhelmed, unable to manage her feelings as well as she had previously. She will find herself brought to tears a bit more easily. She will snap or even yell at a much lesser offense. She is fundamentally more reactive than she was previously.

Concentration

Perimenopausal Initiation also brings an increase in distractibility and forgetfulness. Some women begin to see the first signs of losing a train of thought, walking into a room only to forget what they were going to do or finding a need to keep a calendar or checklist. These minimal shifts may be infrequent enough or minor enough that they are easily explained away by a busy day or lack of sleep.

For most women, in Perimenopausal Initiation, these changes may be so subtle, they fly right under the radar. They may only momentarily have a thought asking themselves why they are so: irritable, anxious, jumpy or cranky and then dismiss it as "nothing." Other women will not take note of these differences at all. Sometimes it is the family members that may begin noticing slight variations in the way the Stage I woman reacts or responds. A child may ask, "Mom, why do you look so mad?" Mom may be surprised, deny being "mad' but be perplexed that she does feel a certain emotional discomfort, with no understanding as to why.

Libido

Stage I may also bring about the first signs of declining libido. Again, this change may be nearly imperceptible. Women interpret their less reliable sex drive as being a function of the increasing frustration they may feel with their children or husbands. When she is not excited by his invitation for sex she may truly believe it is because of the dirty underwear he left of the floor, the dishes not placed in the dishwasher or that he did not help the children with their homework.

Stage II: Emotional Disruption

When a woman progresses through the stage of Emotional Disruption, she begins to consciously realize that she is feeling somewhat distressed. Her emotional "fuse" is shorter; she feels much more reactive to the daily stresses and challenges of life. She finds she has less patience for her job, children and her husband. The woman in the stage of Emotional Disruption will find herself rolling her eyes and impatiently muttering under her breath, "It's just easier to do it myself," when her husband does not do things the way she wants them done. This woman will find herself simmering when she sees the muddy footprints from the dog or is interrupted during dinner by a solicitor calling. Her general state is more anxious. This was not how she would have responded before. A Stage II woman's previous mode of handling trying situations might have been a sigh and a bit of resignation that it certainly is a challenge to run a household! Now it is as if the volume on everything has been turned up a notch or two. The difference between Stage I, Perimenopausal Initiation and Stage II, Emotional Disruption, is that in Stage II, Emotional Disruption, the symptoms are more intense and more constant whereas in Stage I, Perimenopausal Initiation, they are more reactive in the moment and not as constant.

Menstruation

Physiologically, the woman in Emotional Disruption will still have regular periods, but she may, upon examination, realize that the cycle fluctuates a bit. She may menstruate a day or two early or late on occasion. Her flow may seem a bit heavier and she will probably experience more cramps. The changes in her cycle will be subtle enough that she will probably attribute the fluctuation to being under more stress or having a lack of sleep, not as a sign of perimenopause being under way. I have heard from a number of women, that they begin to have some cramping mid-cycle, during the ovulation phase of the cycle, some even reporting significant pain.

PMS

The premenstrual phase in the monthly cycle of women in Emotional Disruption will begin to become increasingly difficult, emotionally. Women, who are *not* prone to emotional distress premenstrually, may begin to experience, for the first time, a disruption in their sense of wellbeing. Women who *are* experienced with the typical moodiness of PMS will endure an increased lability of moods. It is in the premenstrual phase that it is most likely the women will start to become aware that things are different. Premenstrual symptoms begin backing up from the few days before menses, to a week to two weeks before. Cramps are more uncomfortable, bloating is more noticeable and breast swelling and tenderness can start to become painful. Women in Emotional Disruption may attribute an increase in moodiness to the increased physical discomfort. While increased discomfort certainly adds to increased moodiness, the emotional changes these women are experiencing are also directly resulting from the hormonal changes happening in their bodies.

Moods

Women in this stage of perimenopause find it more and more difficult to cope with everyday stressors. The overall increase in anxiety they experience is interfering with daily functioning. Women are increasingly aware that their own feelings and reactivity are somewhat alien. Cheryl, in Chapter 7, is a great example of how a woman in the stage of Emotional Disruption can feel off-kilter without understanding that she has begun the hormonal changes of perimenopause. What Cheryl was *aware* of feeling, was stressed and uncomfortable with her life. Her feelings were subtle but pervasive. Feeling overwhelmed, as Cheryl did, is commonplace for women in this stage.

Concentration

The distractibility and forgetfulness that began in Perimenopausal Initiation are now becoming more intrusive. If we recall our forgetful ladies from Chapter 9—Suzie who put the orange juice in the cupboard, Cindy who gave her weekly dinner budget to the locksmith, and Amy (from Chapter 7) who chilled her keys in the refrigerator—we can see how disruptive these lapses in concentration can be. Unfortunately, this adds to the angst of the woman in Emotional Disruption. Many women become convinced they are suffering from dementia, Alzheimer's Disease, Attention Deficit Disorder or brain tumors when these particular challenges gain momentum in this stage of perimenopause. The anxiety associated with the frustration and concern over this absentmindedness can become enormous and exacerbate the anxiety that is already present.

When women in Emotional Disruption encounter such restlessness that has no apparent reason, they begin to look for explanations for their emotional angst. For example, a typical scenario would involve a woman coming in after a demanding day at work. She sees toys scattered across the floor, food left out on the kitchen counter and quickly assesses that the children's homework has not been done. In times prior to the hormonal changes of perimenopause, she would take a moment, catch her breath and shift into "mom mode," organizing, straightening and barking commands to establish order and responsibility in the household. When in Emotional Disruption, she will encounter the same chaos, feel completely overwhelmed, anxious and even a sinking feeling of depression. Rather than rolling up her sleeves and jumping in, she feels herself curl up inside and wants to go lock herself in her bedroom, pulling the covers over her head. She is on the verge of tears from the frustration. She may begin screaming and blaming. The message playing in her mind is that if everyone would just do as they were supposed to, she would not have to deal with all of this upset. *She is unaware that what has changed is her internal state, not the external circumstance.* Catching the next plane to nowhere or dreams of escaping to a private island are a familiar theme in the frustrated and frazzled minds of these women.

Stage III: Turbulence

In the third stage of perimenopause, Turbulence, women are deeply in the throes of their menopausal transition. Simply put, they are in an emotional tornado. Moods now fluctuate widely, frequently and unpredictably. No longer are mood fluctuations only a part of the premenstrual days. They will be present throughout the monthly cycle, if there still is a reliable monthly cycle. The emotional chaos is so powerful, it is not only a disruption in daytime hours, but it invades sleep and dreams. Turbulence is the stage of perimenopause when women often feel that they no longer know themselves. They may cry or rage at the drop of a hat.

More about Tara

If we recall Tara, from Chapter Four, the medical health professional, who was having problems with flooding, we can see that she was well into perimenopause. Tara dismally relayed the story that while in her office early one morning, she received two consecutive phone calls from people requesting changes in their appointments. While appointment changes were always annoying, on this particular day, Tara hung up the phone and burst into tears. Tara, who prided herself on being the consummate, cool-headed professional, was shocked at her own reaction. The only consolation was that thankfully, she was, alone when it happened!

Tara's story shows us the unpredictable, sometimes spontaneous, shift in emotions, characteristic of women in Turbulence. Physiologically, estrogen levels vary widely on a continual basis. Progesterone levels are at a low ebb leaving women without the calming shield to protect against the vacillating estrogen. Most women notice changes in their cycles. Some women may skip periods while others may only see small changes in the regularity or the flow. What is absolute is that women in Turbulence are recognizable to themselves and to others as emotionally different.

Anxiety

When women enter into Stage III, Turbulence, they experience a significant increase in their levels of anxiety, far more than in Stage II, Emotional Disruption. When reflecting on Christine, whom we met in Chapter 6, the woman who loved to travel but suffered panic attacks on a vacation with her husband, we see how anxiety levels can skyrocket, almost without reason. Women who never before had an inclination towards anxiety may find themselves having panic attacks.

In Turbulence, anxiety also works its way into the nighttime hours. This is the stage of perimenopause when women begin to have the most trouble sleeping. Initially, the sleep disruption is solely due to the hormonally induced anxiety. After nights of restless sleep and exhausting days that follow, the degrading sleep patterns described in Chapter 9 may set in; sleepless nights increase the anxiety that there will be more sleepless nights, which in turn *causes* a worsening of insomnia.

Many women find the unpredictable, often extreme anxiety states of Stage III, Turbulence the most difficult part of perimenopause, especially when the anxiety sets off panic attacks. In rare cases, the anxiety may reach phobic proportions. This will be more likely when a woman has a prior history of suffering from anxiety. Some of the more common phobias and severe anxiety states in Turbulence include obsessive/compulsive behaviors, agoraphobia, and claustrophobia. Rather than suffer with such a severe disruption to healthy living, women experiencing such symptoms would need to seek psychological or medical intervention.

Depression

The sister emotion to intense anxiety in the stage of Turbulence, is depression. Women, who were never prone to depression may find themselves fighting despair. The increase in depression during this stage of perimenopause is notable. Many women awaken in the morning already feeling defeated. Getting out of bed and into the shower may take a Herculean effort. Once again, this was not typical prior to perimenopause. A simple disappointment, an argument with her husband, a reproach from her boss may evoke tears or even a total meltdown. We can revisit Sari, from Chapter 1, who desperately tried to figure out why she was so weepy when she had the "picture perfect" life.

Many women report feeling miserable with just about everything in their lives during this stage of perimenopause. The simplest thing things may feel overwhelming. What was easily accomplished previously may become nearly impossible. Since depression creates fatigue, these women will not only feel extreme sadness, but will also experience profound exhaustion. Together, these feelings make functioning profoundly difficult.

When in Turbulence, the desire to find reasons to explain one's mood is more intense than in Stage II, Emotional Disruption. This confusion has the potential of becoming extremely destructive in a woman's life. Many women look for explanations for their internal distress in the behaviors of those closest to them, often their husbands'. The routines or flaws that spouses have always exhibited, now become intolerable. The messy husband's sloppy habits now become an explanation for a woman's irritability or reason for a mean-spirited backlash. The cognizant woman will be surprised at some of the words and hostilities that have come out of her mouth. Self-restraint is in short supply in woman in Turbulence.

Women who do not have this level of self-awareness may continue to blame their distress on others. In extreme cases, women begin to contemplate separation or even divorce as they reaffirm in their minds their husbands being the cause of all of their misery. For this reason, it is unwise for women to make rash decisions in this state of their perimenopause. What is completely intolerable now, may become a simple annoyance once they are in Quietitude, the final stage of perimenopause.

Dreaming

When the intense emotionality of Turbulence enters the night-time arena, it will be reflected in sleep and in dreams. Women often report awakening in the middle of the night with severe anxiety—even panic attacks. Sometimes this is a result of the hormonally driven emotions; other times a result of the hormonally driven dreams. We saw in Chapter 9 the progression of dreams that Mindy had as she progressed through perimenopause. It was as she entered Turbulence that her dreams became very disturbing showing her torment over her bloated, yet empty womb.

Mindy had another disturbing dream in Turbulence. This time she dreamed she had her period and was bleeding uncontrollably. She desperately needed surgery and was searching for her mother and her sisters to help her. The dream was very intense and emotional. She was distraught and frightened. No one was available to save her, to fix her. In the end, she managed to handle it all herself and the crisis passed.

Mindy's dream illustrates the depth and breadth of the emotional fervor in Turbulence. *The conscious anxieties, fears and sadness are tied directly to the subconscious and unconscious dream states.* On all levels Mindy's emotions were chaotic and intense. We can also see that Mindy, in this dream, is approaching Stage IV, Quietitude. The peaceful resolution she accomplishes by herself is a clear indicator that some of the disturbing emotional tides are ready to begin finding a quieter rhythm.

PMS

The premenstrual phase is extremely difficult in Turbulence. The premenstrual mood swings, notably anxiety and depression, are extraordinarily intense. This is made more complicated when the menstrual cycles are irregular because a woman does not know when she is premenstrual. Some conceptualize depression as the antithesis of anxiety, but certainly in these variable hormonal times, they live side by side in unending disharmony. Often the presence of one will exacerbate the intensity of the other. The feelings of anxiety or the presence of panic attacks can feel so unsettling to a woman, that she finds herself feeling depressed. When she feels limited, nervous and out of sorts, her mood downshifts. Similarly, when a woman feels depressed a significant amount of time, she may become anxious, wondering how and when she will feel like her former self and if she will ever be able to resume her responsibilities. The emotional chaos she is experiencing is not unlike that of puberty; no one knows what to expect, other than that it will be unpredictable and seemingly irrational.

This is the disarming characteristic of Turbulence. What we know about ourselves, no longer applies. Before perimenopause we have a basic knowledge of what we like or dislike, what calms us or agitates us, what we are inured to or sensitive to. When we enter Turbulence, there are no rules; history does not apply. It is akin to being adrift in the ocean during a storm where the wind and the waves buffet us about in any direction.

Stage IV: Quietude

Just as the ocean calms after the storm, so does the perimenopausal woman attain quiescence after turbulence. Turbulence seems like it is a never-ending nightmare. Not only does it end, but the "after" is even better than the "before." Hormonally, in the stage of Quietude, estrogen levels have become more stable, humming at a low ebb. There is a much smaller disparity now between estrogen and progesterone. While menses may still continue, there is no longer a monthly cycle. Several months may be skipped between periods.

In the emotional realm, women feel a sense of completeness and tranquility. Anxiety and depression recede to a level more reminiscent of the pre-perimenopausal period-that of the early to mid-thirties. Focus and concentration, while not returning entirely to pre-perimenopausal levels, approach those levels.

Women in Stage IV, Quietude have survived a difficult journey ripe with changes that ran through every fiber of who they were, both physiologically and psychologically. Disrupting life issues were confronted, because they had to be. Women in Turbulence do not have the option of ignoring issues because their emotions force them to the surface. Whether the outcome was good or bad, was planned or a surprise, there is a sense of having closure—having survived. While Quietude certainly brings a significant reduction in unpleasant emotions, women will continue to have periodic bursts of emotional unpredictability. These outbursts will be more similar to the intensity of the emotions in Emotional Disruption than those in Turbulence. Once in Quietude, these bursts feel like the aberration, rather than the rule.

Table 10-1
Psychological Stages of Perimenopause

	Stage I	Stage II	Stage III	Stage IV
Name	Perimenopausal Initiation	Emotional Disruption	Turbulence	Quietude
Onset	Middle to late thirties, early forties	Early to middle forties	Middle to late forties	Late forties to early fifties
Menstrual cycle	No noticeable change, but some cycles are anovulatory	Monthly cycles with some changes in bleeding patterns	Cyclic variability with decreasing predictability, long and short cycle length	Skipped cycles to ceasing of menstruation
Flow	Primarily unchanged	Increased	Unpredictable-may be heavy or light	Absent, spotting or flooding
Ovulation	Occasional anovulatory cycles	Decreasing frequency of ovulation	Infrequent ovulation-may have severe cramping mid-cycle	Rare to never
Vasomotor symptoms	Minimal to no symptoms-may occasionally appear in PMS phase of cycle	VMS begin to disrupt sleep-primarily in the PMS phase of cycle and during menstruation	VMS become intrusive and may appear throughout the cycle-day and night	VMS may become extremely disruptive to day and nighttime functioning and eventually ease

PMS	Mild worsening	Moderate worsening	Severe	Mild to absent
Moods	Slightly lower threshold for tolerating stress, occasional depression before menses	Even lower threshold for stress, more intense reactivity.	Moods fluctuate dramatically and unpredictably throughout the cycle, high anxiety and depression	Increasing sense of tranquility and empowerment, sense of new beginnings
Cognition	Increased distractibility and forgetfulness	Intrusive and noticeable lapses of concentration	Severe episodes of forgetfulness and lack of concentration, disturbing dreams increase	Dramatic reduction in forgetfulness, increased cognition and concentration

Table 10-1 illustrates the physiological and psychological symptoms of perimenopause and shows how they exert their influence throughout each of the psychological stages of perimenopause. Once again, we can use Mindy, from Chapter 9, as an example of how women may experience the psychological stages of perimenopause.

Mindy had enormous difficulty with her loss of fertility when her child-rearing years were ending. We saw in the sequence of dreams Mindy had, how her emotional struggle was resolved as she progressed through the stages of perimenopause. Initially, in Perimenopausal Initiation, Mindy relived her wonderful pregnancies and birth of her children. As she progressed into Emotional Disruption, she had intense dreams of giving birth to substitutes (kittens and puppies) for children. The disconcerting sense of these dreams is characteristic of the stage of Emotional Disruption.

Next, Mindy began to dream of empty pregnancies. The intense emotion, the anxious sense Mindy felt and the need to be "done" show us that Mindy was in Turbulence. Finally, Mindy came to a satisfying acceptance of where she was in life…and who she was now—the hallmark of Quietude. Many women will feel stronger, more confident and have a better sense of who they are in Quietude. Once again, they feel they know themselves and can be comfortable anticipating their feelings and reactions. We can easily see there is a stark improvement in how a woman feels living life, from the emotional turmoil of Turbulence to the calm acceptance of Quietude.

Chapter Eleven

The Birth of Anxiety

erimenopause gives rise to significant changes throughout a woman's body. We have learned about the many hormonal changes and how these affect multiple systems in the body. These hormonal changes also bring about many neurochemical changes that impact women's moods, emotions and psychological states. Some of this was discussed earlier when we looked at the changes that take place in the brains of females in puberty and in the perimenopausal period.

These enormous changes happening at this perimenopausal phase of life create an emotional crossroads for many women. The physiology of perimenopause tends to lower the threshold for tolerating difficult issues that may have been easily manageable in the past. This becomes a time of reckoning in that so many unresolved emotional and psychological issues from the past begin to well up and "overflow their banks." Anxiety can be a prickly thorn complicating the lives of women approaching or already in the throes of perimenopause.

Working Mothers

Women today have fallen into a pattern of always putting others first. The needs of the family take precedence over their own needs. Many women today are not just raising families and taking care of the household, they are also working outside of the home. The entrance of the woman into the workplace has had the effect of multiplying women's chores, responsibilities and stresses.

The working mom finds herself up at 5:00 in the morning, beginning the various chores of getting meals made, children ready for school and the house tidied so she can be at work by 8:00 or 9:00 A.M. After working a full day, she rushes home to pick up the children from aftercare, get dinner on the table, help the children with the homework while being filled in on children's peer and school issues as well as her husband's workday, and then she begins making or returning phone calls. Only once the children are put to bed, can she then clean up the house, throw in a load or two of laundry, pay some bills and begin to prepare for the next day.

Somewhere around midnight, she collapses into bed, exhausted. There is no time during the day for her to unwind and relax. There is no time for her to sit with her own thoughts and explore herself, her relationships and her future. She is deprived of nurturing from others but primarily from nurturing herself. This pattern goes on day after day, year after year with increasing exhaustion and stress for the woman. Becky is a perfect example of the modern day working mom.

Becky's Distress

Becky, her husband and two young children bought a new house in the perfect neighborhood. The school system was excellent; there was an active community and an abundance of nice families with young children around. Although the home was at the upper limits of what Becky and her husband could afford, they felt it was a wise move when all was considered. Becky was willing to continue at her part time job in order to afford this opportunity.

After moving in, Becky jumped right into getting involved in the community. She joined the temple, volunteering for several committees, joined the Parent Teacher's Association (PTA) at the school and worked hard to meet other women to develop friendships. So what if the house did not get furnished? All was going well. Then Becky's husband had a salary reduction at his job. Now Becky had to begin working full time.

The first time I met Becky, she had deep dark circles under her eyes, her face was pale and drawn and she was on the verge of utter exhaustion. She was taking medication for severe acid reflux and another for anxiety. She had been working full time for several months. She was afraid to ask for too much from her husband because she was concerned that his ego was still fragile from the situation at his job. She did not want to make him feel emasculated by asking him to do "women's work." Instead, she did it all. She made the children's breakfasts and dinners and packed their school lunches. Since she had to be at work at 8:00 AM, she was typically awake before 6:00. Becky, being a very conscientious and involved mother, was always involved in her children's activities and kept a running contact with the parents of her children's friends.

Since Becky did not want to disappoint the women she had committed herself to in the PTA and other committees she had joined, she continued with these activities as well. It was not unusual for Becky to be finishing a task or project after midnight, long after her family was sound asleep. Becky bemoaned that she could not remember the last time she was in bed before midnight. Becky was living the mistake of considering everyone else's needs to the exclusion of her own. She was on a collision course with disaster if she did not start to make some changes, and soon!

Over-Scheduling

The example of Becky shows a typical pattern for the working mom. Now let us add to this all of the extras that women have to incorporate into their lives, whether or not they work outside of the home. Over-scheduling is a problem that often overwhelms women. Schedules have become very complex and demanding in our highly pressured culture. Parents, children and schools all induce children to be involved in numerous extracurricular activities.

Today, children are involved in more than one sport, sometimes three or four. They take karate lessons, dance lessons, art lessons, academic tutoring and go to religious school. They have birthday parties to go to and like to have play dates. One exhausted mother of three told me each of her children was always involved in two sports. She had to chauffeur each of them to all of their practices and games. It was her personal goal never to miss a game. Imagine her stress level when the games overlapped! She would frantically rush from one game to the other, often at different schools, to see part of the game in which each child was playing. If this was not enough, she also got her children to religious lessons after school.

After years of maintaining this level of stress, exhaustion and anxiety, as she headed into her late forties, this mom suffered from an emotional and physical collapse.

Elderly Parents

Now, ladies, does this cover the total stress load under which we exist? I have only begun to outline what women deal with today. Because women now tend to marry later and start their families later, they are often faced with elderly, sick parents while their children are still young. Many couples have to negotiate medical care, transportation and finances for their older parents. In addition, adult children often feel obligated to help their elderly or feeble parents maintain independent living so the women must manage their daily needs. This places an enormous strain on an already strained situation. Oftentimes a woman feels responsible for taking care of a parent who has been widowed or divorced and begins to have trouble caring for him- or herself. Knowing that she is already overloaded and close to her breaking point, a woman will rationalize that since the parent always took care of her, it is now her obligation to return the favor.

In some situations a decision is made to move an elderly parent into the family home, believing it would be an easy and sensible solution for all involved. Unfortunately, it is not that simple. An adult parent has his or her own ideas regarding how to run his or her life. Adding a formerly independent adult into your household typically brings a very bumpy transition for the whole family. As the woman of the house, you are accustomed to running your household your way. The more demanding the schedules of the family, the less negotiating room and desire there will be to accommodate that parent. In my practice, I have come to see this as the most stressful of the possible options for women who have elderly parents that are compromised in some way.

Renee's Resentment

Renee had two toddlers, worked full time and was barely able to keep things running smoothly. Her life was a constant juggling act to get her children into daycare on time so she could get to work. She constantly felt the pressure of home while at work because her workday had to end when daycare was over. Her job involved a lot of travel, which added additional strain to both her husband's and her schedules.

Renee was in her early forties when her mother was widowed. Unfortunately, when all was settled, it was determined that Renee's mother was not in good financial shape after her husband died. Nor was she very happy about living alone. Although Renee had two siblings, the mother's care fell on Renee's shoulders. Initially, she was making frequent visits to her mother, inviting her mother to her home, helping financially, (which did cause a strain on Renee's budget), and taking mom on her errands. Renee was already stretched beyond reason and this was bringing her to a breaking point.

Renee and her husband decided to invite mom to live with them. It would save money, ease Renee's running around and she could keep a close eye on mom.

Unfortunately, things did not go as planned. Mom began to become dependent on Renee as her outlet for her grief and anger at her situation. Her distress precluded her from helping Renee with some of her burdens. Mom's health began to deteriorate and now Renee had to add to her schedule taking her mother to numerous doctor appointments. Renee began to suffer with declining health. Her menstrual cycles began to shift and she started developing debilitating migraines. Renee began to resent her mother's presence in her home and life. Mom resented Renee's lack of empathy. Renee and her husband began arguing frequently because of the intrusiveness of the mother and the overall increase of tension in the household. The situation came to a head when Renee and her husband began to talk about divorce.

Even when the parent is not brought in to live with their children, taking care of them in their own dwelling can be a challenge, too. In some situations, decisions must be made about moving parents to another living arrangement that is more appropriate for their needs. Some elderly parents may be quite willing to make this transition but others may be enormously resistant. In either case, the job of finding the right place, making the arrangements and dismantling the parents' former abode often falls on their children. Whether this is a woman's own parents or her husband's, much of the stress will wind up on her. Once the transition is agreed upon and made, there is continued responsibility and stress in seeing to it that the parents are happy and well cared for.

There is, of course is a much greater challenge when the family decides to maintain the elderly parent in their original home. In this case, adult children feel nearly constant anxiety regarding how well the parent is able to care for him- or herself. Knowing that an elderly parent who may have some health challenges or has never lived on their own is now managing their own lives in their own dwelling, leaves their loved ones in a position of tremendous responsibility and continuous concern.

Never Say "No": Women in their Community

As we saw earlier, in the story of Becky, many women just do not know how to say "no." Whenever they are asked to help out, join a committee, run a fundraiser or help a friend or neighbor, they feel compelled to do whatever has been asked of them. In our culture, women are socialized to be pleasers. They also have hormonally induced brain structures to incline them to be nurturers. [99]

Women do not typically consider how much they are already obligated to do before accepting yet another obligation. When asked to help out, they feel they must accept, regardless of what sort of strain this may place on them. A woman, as opposed to a man, will be more concerned with how the other will feel if she says "no" rather than how she, herself, will feel if she says "yes."' This is not only an issue for requests that come from outside of the family, such as church or temple groups, school associations, friends and community organizations, but also from immediate family members—the children and husbands.

How often do we see women who work full time also taking on all of the household responsibilities? How many working women are unwilling to ask their husbands to take on the task of doing the laundry, housecleaning or cooking? How typical is it for the husband to buy the birthday gift for children's parties or the holiday gifts for teachers, family or friends? Which parent is in contact with the teachers or the school if the child is having problems? Who takes the children to buy clothes? Who accompanies the husband in buying clothes?

This is not meant to imply that men do not participate in running a home and maintaining a household. Many husbands and fathers are more and more willing to share in the duties of the home. The difficulty for women is that they and their spouses share a perspective that the men are helping their wives when they help out at home rather than viewing these as mutual responsibilities that should be divided fairly. Hence, the onus is on the woman to ask for the help; he then, is doing her the favor by providing it.

Such a situation creates enormous anxiety for women. They feel indebtedness when asking for and getting their spouses' participation. The dynamic between husband and wife becomes such that she must be cautious about how much she requests and must be grateful for what he provides. He, after all, may become resentful if she asks for too much. This places enormous, relentless strain on women. Some women wind up deciding that it is all just easier to do it themselves. These are the women who end up like Becky, exhausted, stressed and overwhelmed.

Chapter Twelve

Stress Becomes Anxiety

The relentless daily stresses that women experience in their forties begin to build on one another until they reach a crisis point. Stress, which is an externally induced tension, is the precursor to anxiety, a very disquieting internal sense of overwhelming fear or apprehension. Physical and emotional stress and resulting exhaustion, along with hormonal shifts, wear women down to the degree that they are vulnerable to suffering from anxiety.

Let us stop and think for a moment about what we have just learned. Women are overburdened and overstressed. This wears on their adrenal glands. The adrenal glands are tiny hormone-producing glands that sit on top of the kidneys. They impact every organ, gland and tissue in the body by producing over fifty different hormones including cortisol, noradrenalin, estrogen and testosterone. Healthy functioning of the adrenal glands cannot be underestimated. They support immune system functioning by their anti-oxidant and anti-inflammatory actions, they regulate blood sugar, fluid balance, the utilization of carbohydrates and fats and are instrumental in healthy thyroid functioning (see Appendix II for more information).

As perimenopause progresses into menopause, it is the adrenal glands that become the primary source for the production of sex hormones in the body. Years of high stress levels begin to exhaust the adrenal glands. This creates a domino effect in the body that compromises the healthy functioning of all of these systems, eventually leaving the body with fewer resources to recover from the physiological impacts of perimenopause and the emotional distress from years of pushing beyond one's reasonable limits. Together, this worsens the symptoms of stress while challenging the body's ability to recover.

Typically, in our culture, the most stressful period of a woman's life seems to be the period lasting from the late thirties into the late forties or early fifties. For women who are mothers, this is when the logistical and emotional demands of raising children—particularly adolescents and teens—may intensify. Often this occurs in a context of rising expenses. Children are involved in many costly activities, mortgage and car payments must be made and parents are trying to figure out how they are going to manage the exorbitant costs for college. Many women of this age are either continuing to work or returning to work. Throughout all of this, the hormonal changes of perimenopause are exerting their influence.

An added challenge during these years is that many marriages lose their bloom as couples become entrenched in the tedious everyday tasks of raising a family, working and taking care of the household. Romance between spouses begins to feel like the intangible memory of something lovely but in the past. Meanwhile, the exhausted adrenal glands begin to trigger irregular sleep patterns, a compromised immune system, a reduction in vitality and significant fatigue. All of these stressors, combined with the hormonal effects of perimenopause, can overload a woman's ability to cope and can result in overwhelming anxiety.

If you have ever had the experience of driving your car when another car suddenly swerves in front of you, you are familiar with the sudden flood of adrenaline that spills into your bloodstream. You are aware of your heart pounding and that sense of every fiber in your body being on alert. There is no collision, so there you sit in your car, immobile, trying to calm down. Assuming you are not prone to a violent episode of road rage, you have no outlet for the overpowering state of anxiety your body is in. It may take some time for your body to return to a semi-relaxed state but even then, you may feel an increase of anxiety every time you see another car getting a bit too close to you. This is a very concrete way of understanding how the physiological response becomes a psychological issue. The external stressor becomes internal anxiety.

When living a very stressful life filled with responsibilities and obligations that utilize the bulk of your time and energy, you are living with a constant stream of stressors that have no physical outlet, as in the example above. The physiological cycle begins with the secretion of the stress hormones. The overproduction of the stress hormones creates the range of emotions described above.

Women become so accustomed to experiencing this perpetual high level of stress that they often are unaware that there is a constant knot in their gut or that their jaws are continually clenched. This begins to take a tremendous toll on them and those around them. Before long, anxiety has become an ever-present phenomenon. This is when the external experience of stress becomes the internal state of anxiety. Anxiety is present when the uncomfortable feelings of tension, worry, sleeplessness, weight gain or loss, fears and irritability become continuously present rather than temporarily elicited in response to a particular event.

Chapter Thirteen

Differentiating Between Anxiety Disorders

Generalized Anxiety Disorder

What actually is anxiety? Anxiety is a group of disorders that include phobias, Obsessive-Compulsive Disorder, stress disorders and panic disorders. It is present in twice as many women as men.[100] The type of anxiety typically referred to in everyday language is Generalized Anxiety Disorder (GAD). When a person is suffering from GAD, they feel both psychological and somatic symptoms commonly associated with feeling nervous or stressed, that of muscle tension, tightening in the throat, edginess, worrying, diarrhea, constipation, nausea, vomiting, headaches, migraines, and excessive sweating.[101] Usually those with somatic symptoms also have a high degree of psychological symptoms. These symptoms can be so severe they can disrupt an individual's sense of wellbeing, productivity and at their most severe, even their ability to function.

There is an enormous range of symptoms in people with Anxiety Disorders. Often people are not even aware that what they are suffering from is anxiety, more so when they focus only on their somatic symptoms.

A State of Conflict

One young woman came to my office after an exhaustive series of medical tests. She had been exceedingly nauseous and began vomiting regularly for close to a year. She could not keep down any food and was losing weight and strength at an alarming rate. She was on disability because she had deteriorated to a level that precluded her from working or caring for herself. Her gastrointestinal system was tested with every medical test known to the medical community. After being hospitalized, medicated, tested for allergies and put on various diets, it was all to no avail. She had been a patient of the medical community for nearly a year with no improvement. During that time she and her doctors assumed the problem was a medical one.

In my first session with her, it became immediately apparent that this woman was in a terrible state of conflict in her personal life. She had made choices that were completely at odds with who she was and how she wanted to live her life. All of her symptoms were a result of anxiety. In our work together she learned how to take control of her life and her choices.

In a matter of weeks, the vomiting lessened. It was only a few months before it stopped completely. She began eating and gaining weight and for the first time in a long time this young woman began to see herself as a participant in life instead of an observer. Within eight months she had returned fully and completely to a healthy, satisfying existence. Her somatic symptoms were gone and her anxiety was reduced to a tolerable, level in which she was able to resume normal functioning.

While all people experience some level of worry or anxiety at one time or another, the degree of worry that people with GAD experience is excessive. It becomes an impediment to functioning in social or occupational areas and causes significant distress. This excessive worrying can become irrational and can begin to generalize. Often it can have a domino effect where the anxiety begins to create unpleasant situations that in turn create more anxiety.

For example, one woman, Gloria, was feeling a substantial amount of anxiety. Gloria began to worry that people at work might notice. The more worried she became, the more difficult it was for her to concentrate. She began to avoid being around her coworkers, believing that her feelings were very obvious to others. Because of this expanding worry Gloria made a couple of errors at work. This, in turn, heightened her anxiety even more.

It is easy to see how untreated anxiety can spiral out of control. People suffering with this type of anxiety are prone to sleep disturbances that may be in the form of falling asleep, staying asleep or having restless sleep. This, too, becomes part of the expanding nature of anxiety. The more sleep deprived one becomes, the more vulnerable they become to experiencing mood disorders, including depression and anxiety. The sleep disturbance combined with the strain and tension they continually feel may result in even greater fatigue and in difficulty concentrating.

Anxious Lucille

Another example of the impact anxiety can have is that of Lucille. Lucille, a middle aged woman, newly retired, believed that life could not be any better. She had a nice pension, was happily married and looking forward to being out of the "rat race." Within a short time, Lucille began to have some trouble sleeping. Before long, Lucille was suffering from chronic insomnia. She began to feel incessant worry about issues that had never before concerned her. Her mouth was constantly dry and she always had "a lump in her throat." She began to focus excessively on somatic issues. Every ache or pain sent her running to the doctor. Even after the doctors concluded that she was fine, Lucille continued to worry and lose sleep. Completely convinced that her doctors were "missing something" and that there must be some disease lurking within, she was resistant to therapy. Eventually, at the insistence of her sister, Lucille came to see me. Lucille was suffering from GAD. It took a bit of work before she came to understand the very powerful effects that anxiety can have on the body.

Virtually any illness can be made worse when anxiety gets a foothold and many illnesses may actually be caused by it. Women in their twenties, thirties and early forties seem to be more vulnerable to suffering from GAD than are men. In one study up to five percent of people had GAD, with 50 to 60 percent being female.[102]

Often the medical community misdiagnoses those suffering with GAD because they focus only on the somatic symptoms that are present. This leaves the individual with treatment for the symptoms without ever finding the cause. When the treatment is stopped, the symptoms return.

The stressors that contribute to anxiety in each stage of life tend to be somewhat unique to that stage. Women in their twenties are more likely to find that their stresses are from issues surrounding beginning careers, starting serious relationships, establishing their own homes and managing independence. Stresses in the thirties focus on beginning families, raising children, solidifying marriages and family and juggling household, family and work responsibilities. The forties includes many of the stresses of the thirties but women also begin to feel the angst of seeing their roles beginning to change as their children get older. They may begin to experience health-related problems in themselves, spouses, family and friends for the first time. In the early to mid-forties changing hormones are becoming a factor in increasing anxiety. In the middle forties financial concerns loom larger as retirement becomes a visible reality.

The later forties and the fifties bring a major shift in a how a woman identifies herself. This is often one of the more challenging stressors of adulthood as women enter the empty nest period. They have to renegotiate their relationships with their husbands as they find a new identity, meaning and purpose for themselves. They struggle with the concerns and demands of aging parents while simultaneously they are confronting the loss of their fertility. Each phase of life with its unique challenges and stressors provides its own contribution to women's vulnerability to suffering from GAD.

Adjustment Disorder with Anxiety

An Adjustment Disorder is diagnosed in a symptomatic individual who has been exposed to a specific psychosocial stressor within the prior three months. There are emotional or behavioral symptoms that indicate a level of distress that is disproportionate to what would typically occur with that stressor. The individual with Adjustment Disorder with Anxiety feels the anxiety symptoms we saw in GAD; worry, tension, fear, somatic complaints, insomnia, etc. She will also experience a serious disruption in social, occupational or academic functioning, similar to what we see with GAD.

The difference between GAD and an Adjustment Disorder is that an Adjustment Disorder is short-lived, lasting a maximum of six months after exposure to the stressor, and there is a specific stressor. In GAD, this is not the case. If the stressor is ongoing, or in the event there are a series of stressors, the Adjustment Disorder may last longer than six months.[103]

While perimenopausal women may receive this diagnosis, it would not be a direct result of the hormonal changes they are experiencing. A woman who is already vulnerable to emotional distress because of her physiological difficulties may find herself less able to cope with a specific psychosocial stressor. This may increase the likelihood of her succumbing to an Adjustment Disorder, but it would not be the direct cause.

Anxiety Disorder Due to a General Medical Condition

Another common Anxiety Disorder that appears in women in their forties and fifties is *Anxiety Disorder Due to a General Medical Condition*. This type of anxiety is one that is caused by a variety of medical conditions including, but not limited to metabolic disorders and endocrine disorders.

The symptoms of Anxiety Disorder Due to a General Medical Condition are similar to the symptoms of GAD. The excessive worry, feelings of nervousness, muscle tension, tightening in the throat and edginess are symptoms of Anxiety Disorder Due to a General Medical Condition as well as GAD. Both of these anxiety disorders share symptoms of sleep disturbances, trouble with concentration, focusing and exhaustion. Both may include somatic complaints. People with this diagnosis are also prone to the same challenges in functioning in important areas of life such as at work, home or in social situations because of the excessive worrying.[104]

The major difference between these two types of Anxiety Disorders is that Anxiety Disorder Due to a General Medical Condition is an Anxiety Disorder that is unequivocally a result of a medical disorder. It is the medical condition that directly and physiologically creates the Anxiety Disorder. This is not the case with GAD. Although both disorders may have somatic or physiological attributes, it is only in Anxiety Disorder Due to a General Medical Condition that the Anxiety Disorder is caused by a medical condition.

As we have already learned, the changing hormones of perimenopause have been shown to create an increase in anxiety. The associated medical conditions of thyroid dysfunction (see Part III) and adrenal dysfunction can also initiate the onset of an Anxiety Disorder. Thus, there is ample cause to consider Anxiety Disorder Due to a General Medical Condition when diagnosing a perimenopausal woman with an Anxiety Disorder.

If the symptoms are so similar, why make the distinction between these two types of Anxiety Disorders? The reason is that it is critically important for a woman to understand what is happening to her and why. She needs to know if her anxiety is a direct result of the endocrine or metabolic changes happening in her body or if the anxiety is an expression of other unresolved emotional issues that may have been exacerbated by the hormonal changes in her body. If she is treated only for the psychological aspect of her condition, important medical issues may be ignored and neglected.

One example of this is the anxiety associated with vasomotor symptoms in perimenopause. In the early phases of perimenopause, prior to a woman's menstrual period, there often are early morning night sweats. It is believed that these vasomotor symptoms are a function of declining estrogen. Often these early morning sweats are preceded by a combination of anxiety symptoms, including panic, palpitations, nausea, dizziness, anger or feeling faint. When a woman lacks the knowledge of the physiological connection (in this case her declining estrogen) to her psychological feelings, the anxiety may worsen as she searches for and begins to fear the possible explanations for her unpleasant sensations.

Understanding these differences between diagnoses is also important to determine the type of treatment a woman seeks. Treatment of Anxiety Disorder Due to a General Medical Condition may require more of a medical, pharmaceutical or physiological component, in conjunction with psychotherapy, while GAD would require a psychological focus, possibly without the intervention of medical treatment.

Chapter Fourteen
The Face of Anxiety: How the Anxious Woman Appears to Others

ometimes it can be difficult for women to recognize that they are feeling anxiety since feelings of anxiety can masquerade as any number of physical and/or psychological symptoms. What is even more of a challenge is for women to realize how their internal state of anxiety is expressed to those around them. An internally anxious state can be expressed in an infinite number of ways, some of which can be quite destructive. Women have widely varying ways of handling their anxiety. Some may internalize anxious feelings, creating somatic symptoms such as bowel problems, headaches, high blood pressure or lowered immunity. Other women may externalize their anxiety.

One of the more common ways in which anxiety finds its outlet is also one of the most damaging, that of expressed hostility. When a woman finds herself all knotted up inside, with an internal sense of expanding frustration and irritability, she may feel, or her friends, family and coworkers may experience her as being short tempered, extremely reactive or even hostile. Internally she may feel that people are just getting on her nerves. She may recognize feeling edgy but may attribute her edginess to the actions of those around her rather than to an internal state of anxiety. An anxious woman may find herself thinking, "If only my husband would put his underwear in the hamper, I wouldn't be so furious," or, "I wouldn't be screaming if my child would just eat his dinner." It is not that the actions of those around her do not legitimately frustrate her, it is when her reaction is so out of proportion to the offense that it becomes problematic and indicates that something else must be going on.

A woman in this situation frequently will be shocked at what has come out of her own mouth in an unguarded moment. She will find herself overreacting, perhaps screaming at her child for leaving a dirty dish or railing at her husband for ruining her life after committing a minor offense. Coworkers may be intimidated in approaching her when this was never the case prior. Because she does not connect these behaviors with her internal anxious state, those she cares about cannot make that connection either. If she can connect with her internal state of anxiety she can then embark on the journey of uncovering her feelings and then working to alleviate the anxiety.

The kids often get the brunt of this misdirected distress. A child or teen is confused when experiencing anger or hostility from a parent that is out of proportion to the offense. Not understanding that Mom's insides are roiling from an excess of anxiety, the child is likely to interpret Mom's reaction as being either an indication of how Mom really feels about the child or that Mom is arbitrarily over-reactive and hence is not a good barometer for assessing one's own actions.

Imagine a woman like Doris, feeling short tempered, frustrated and impatient from her anxiety. Doris' young son approaches her, whining about what she is cooking for dinner. She initially snaps at him, feeling very overwhelmed and unappreciated. He continues to whine, reacting to her impatience, stating that he just will not eat what she has cooked. In a flash Doris is screaming at him, threatening all sorts of consequences, perhaps even blaming him for her "stress." Internally, she is resisting an urge to fling the dinner in the sink, grab her keys and drive off to who knows where! Somewhere in the back of her mind a little voice is questioning why she has just reacted so strongly. What is going on? She may even experience a pang of guilt as she sees the hurt cross her child's face. This is an unhealthy situation for both of them.

In its most extreme, this dynamic can become the initiator for a breach in the relationship between mother and child. Children require reasonable and predictable reactions and feedback when interacting with their parents in order to make sense of their relationships. When a mother's normal response is biased by her anxiety, the child has no way of assessing what is really happening. When anxiety is significant and prolonged, the children begin to lose more and more objectivity and balance in their relationship with their mother. Mom's responses have become unpredictable and arbitrary.

Most children have the capacity to occasionally pass off Mom's "bizarre" reaction to the fact that Mom is simply in a bad mood. When Mom's state of being becomes irregular on a continual basis, the children become more significantly affected. When a woman is frequently responding to her children with impatience, hostility, nastiness or is constantly snapping, her children will begin to avoid interacting with her. A younger child may begin developing his or her own anxiety in response to Mom's behavior. A teenager may also feel anxiety but more typically will respond with angry, hostile, challenging behavior that may include serious rebellious activities. In all cases, communication is usually challenged and the healthy aspects of the mother-child relationship become jeopardized.

Anxiety, especially in perimenopausal women, can also be a catalyst for marital problems. If she is not aware of the system of anxiety and exhaustion at work inside of her she will often look for reasons outside of herself to explain her predicament. The unrelenting internal pressure that anxious women feel, coupled with the effects of the exhausted adrenal system often lead a woman to look towards her husband either for relief or to blame.

As the anxiety builds over time, a woman, like Doris, will feel increasingly lost, sometimes to the point of desperation. She may broach conversations with her husband in the hope that he may have the answers to her confusion. When he is unable to sort things out or to find the solution, her frustration is likely to turn on him. In her mind, he becomes the reason for her exhaustion and her moodiness. She may find herself angry, displaying challenging and offensive attitudes and behaviors towards him. She enters a cycle of blaming him, becoming disillusioned with their relationship and becoming even more conflicted about her life than before.

As anxiety becomes chronic Doris may find her outlook on life beginning to change in alarming ways. Feeling impatient, frustrated and irritable most of the time begins to take its toll. Her behavior reflects her internal angst and her relationships with those she cares about most, such as her little boy, begin to suffer. As the ripple effect of the symptoms and impact of the anxiety widen, Doris' sleep becomes more disrupted. Her exhausted mental and physical states make it infinitely harder for her to regain her equilibrium. She may begin to feel more insecure as her self-esteem plummets, a result of feeling so inadequate in her most important relationships.

The feedback Doris is receiving from family, friends and coworkers becomes more and more negative. Her drive and initiative begin to decline and her perspective towards life becomes increasingly desolate. This initiates a downward spiral in which life begins to appear overwhelming and hopeless. Before long her ability to function has become compromised. She finds herself avoiding whatever may mobilize her anxiety. An anxious woman often finds her world shrinking as she struggles to find internal peace. It is not uncommon for this type of chronic and or escalating anxiety to eventually lead to depression.

Chapter Fifteen

Treatment Options for Anxiety

$\mathcal{A}$nxiety disorders are distinctive in that they frequently disrupt the wellbeing of those around the anxious individual. Friends and family are typically affected by the symptoms and behaviors of the person suffering from anxiety, especially as the anxious individual tries to manage the unpleasantness of the distress she is experiencing. We have seen how anxious individuals may constrict their worlds, make unreasonable demands or lash out at others in the course of their suffering. For these reasons, the need to treat anxiety goes beyond the benefit of the individual, to those she cares about.

There are many therapies that alleviate anxiety. These therapies include prescribed anxiolytic medications, psychotherapy and eastern therapies such as yoga, acupuncture, breathing and meditation. Currently, the two most popular treatments for anxiety disorders are psychotherapy and anxiolytic medication. The commonly prescribed anxiolytic medications are benzodiazepines (for example Valium, Ativan, and Xanax) and SSRIs (selective serotonin reuptake inhibitors such as Celexa, Paxil, Lexapro and Zoloft).

Anxiolytics

Benzodiazepines are extremely popular because of their effective and immediate relief of anxiety. They facilitate sleep in the anxious individual and can head off and even stop panic attacks. Benzodiazepines also offer a sedating effect for anxiety of a longer duration. The cautionary note for benzodiazepines is that they will impair cognition when taken in higher dosages, are highly addictive and have a rebound effect when they wear off. People who take them for longer than a few weeks will be vulnerable to withdrawal when they are discontinued.

Benzodiazepines are most helpful in the perimenopausal woman when she has episodic anxiety. If she has nights in which she feels unusually stressed and cannot relax to sleep, or awakens and cannot fall back asleep, selected benzodiazepines will work quickly and efficiently to help her relax so she can rest. The same is true for daytime anxiety. When there is a particularly stressful day or event, one of the gentler, slow-acting benzodiazepines will take the edge off. Because of the addictive nature, these are not the best choices for daily long-term use, no matter how anxious the perimenopausal woman is feeling.

SSRIs are classified as antidepressant medications but do have anxiolytic properties. SSRIs require higher doses to treat anxiety than to treat depression. A huge benefit of SSRIs is that they can be used long-term without risk of addiction or dependence. It is not uncommon for the anxious perimenopausal woman to also suffer from depression, so treating anxiety with SSRIs has the added benefits of managing the depression. Recent research has shown another benefit of SSRIs; in perimenopausal women SSRIs are effective in reducing vasomotor events.[105] All of these attributes make this group of medications a good choice for perimenopausal women who are suffering from prolonged anxiety.

Psychotherapy

Traditional individual psychotherapy has proven to be very effective for treating a wide range of anxiety disorders. Psychotherapy helps one identify what events and stimuli provoke anxious feelings and why. Working through such issues allows an individual to find more functional methods of coping with the stressors.

For example, one woman, Trudy, found that nearly every time she had a hot flash, she also had a panic attack. When the hot flashes were severe, she experienced a sensation of claustrophobia. Through psychotherapy, Trudy was able to explore the origins of her anxiety. She gained insight into the role that sickness had played in her childhood. Her mother had suffered with many serious medical problems while Trudy was growing up. Consequently, Trudy, as a child felt frightened and helpless when dealing with all health issues. She experienced overwhelming anxiety as a child that fueled the anxiety she felt as an adult when her own body did not feel right. As she worked through this in therapy, she was able to distinguish the difference between her mother's illness and her own normal transition and explore her current empowered state in contrast to the powerlessness she felt as a child. Eventually, her hot flashes ceased to evoke severe anxiety symptoms.

Psychotherapy will also help the perimenopausal woman identify whether the source of her anxiety is internal or external. Once she can accomplish this, she is less likely to fall into the trap of projecting her anxieties onto those around her. This will allow her to avoid creating the situation in which her distress becomes the catalyst for family dysfunction, as we saw in the case of Doris.

One specific type of psychotherapy that has been very successful in reducing anxiety is cognitive behavioral therapy (CBT).[106] CBT works on the premise that our thoughts control our behaviors and our feelings. By changing the way patients think, via a structured therapeutic program, patients will learn a different way of feeling. With self-reflection gained in therapy she can either manage her anxiety or release it in healthy, functional ways.

Other Therapies

New research indicates promise for hormone therapy. Metabolites of progesterone have shown anxiolytic hypnotic effects similar to that of the benzodiazepines.[107] We have already learned about the sedating, calming effects of progesterone. Hence, it is logical that when perimenopausal women were given bioidentical progesterone supplements, their anxiety was alleviated.[108]

Other effective therapies for reducing anxiety include aerobic exercise, hypnosis, yoga and eating a healthy diet. There is promising research indicating anxiolytic effects in supplements such as kava kava, valerian root, hawthorn, chamomile, passion flower, lemon balm, magnesium[109] and taurine. More details on these treatment options will be given in Chapter 24.

Chapter Sixteen

What is Depression?

epression affects more than 19 million Americans each year, with women being twice as susceptible to experiencing a major depressive episode than men. The gender difference in the prevalence of depression begins early in adolescence, at the start of puberty, suggesting a hormonal influence. Other known contributors to the onset of depression in women beside the hormonal changes of puberty include the hormonal changes of pregnancy and perimenopause, traumatic life events, prior history of depression,[110] substance abuse and personal relationship challenges.

There is also evidence of a higher risk for depression in first degree relatives of those suffering from depression. All of these factors illuminate the role of biological factors, sex hormones and sociocultural factors in the etiology of depression. Depression is considered to be the most burdensome and disabling disease for women, the onset of which peaks in midlife.[111] The risk factors that exist for women will be described below, after a brief outline of several of the more common types of depression.

It is important to know that "depression" is the common term used to represent a wide range of Depressive Disorders. People will often refer to themselves as "depressed" when they are, in reality, simply sad. True depression has specific qualifiers and symptoms, as we will explore shortly. Similar to Anxiety Disorders, there are a number of different levels of severity in the different types of Depressive Disorders. There are also differences in onset, duration and symptoms. We will learn about this and how the various Depressive Disorders have varying characteristics that may make them more or less likely to become exacerbated during periods of great hormonal change that occur in women.

Major Depressive Episode

Suzanne's Depression

Suzanne, a forty-eight year old, single mother of four felt herself decompensating. She was increasingly overwhelmed with her life; raising the children, taking care of the house and working part time to supplement her child support and alimony. She had been struggling with feelings of sadness and being unable to cope since her husband had left her several years before.

As time passed, Suzanne began to falter under the weight of carrying her many burdens. She found it more and more difficult to get up in the mornings. Often she would send the children off to school and climb back into bed, sleeping well into the afternoon. She called out of work so often, she was afraid of losing her job. Suzanne began ordering in food for dinner, a practice she could not afford, because it was too much effort to prepare a meal. She no longer had the energy to see her friends. She had reduced her social contacts to only two of her closest friends, and that was minimal. Her typically immaculate house was dirty and unkempt.

As Suzanne's depression set in, she became less and less interested in life around her. The crisis point came when she could not get out of bed, crying and wondering what the purpose was in

living. Suzanne was suffering from a Major Depressive Episode, a
very severe and debilitating form of depression.

A Major Depressive Episode is diagnosed when an individual is suffering from a sad, depressed mood daily for most of the day combined with a severe decline of interest in daily activities. As we see in Suzanne, this impairment causes a notable challenge for normal functioning and creates a significant amount of distress. The social symptoms that indicate the presence of Major Depressive Episode will be extreme social withdrawal, ambivalence for activities that were previously pleasurable, and a general disinterest in one's life.[112] We saw in the case of Suzanne how even caring for her children became difficult and burdensome.

Appetite Changes

An individual in the throes of a Major Depressive Episode may also experience a marked increase or decrease in appetite accompanied by a significant change in weight. When the appetite is increased, a depressed individual may find herself experiencing food cravings primarily for high carbohydrate or sugary foods. Suzanne could not deny how wrong things were when this typically health-conscious woman found her diet consisting of candy bars. Alternatively the appetite may be diminished, causing the depressed woman to experience eating as being more similar to being force-fed than enjoying a meal.

Sleep Disruption

Another common symptom of Major Depressive Episode is sleep abnormality. This can take the form of hypersomnia, as happened with Suzanne. She slept all night, and then returned to bed to sleep the better part of the day. Conversely, it can present as insomnia. Insomnia falls into three categories: *initial* insomnia, when an individual has trouble falling asleep, *middle* insomnia, characterized by awakening in the middle of the night and having trouble returning to sleep, and *terminal* insomnia, when one awakens too early and cannot return to sleep at all. While both hypersomnia and insomnia are both characteristic of those suffering with depression, insomnia seems to be more troublesome for those suffering with an anxiety disorder while hypersomnia plagues those with depression.

Fatigue

Regardless of how much sleep one gets, individuals suffering from a Major Depressive Episode characteristically suffer from fatigue even in the absence of physical activity. For Suzanne, any small effort required enormous exertion. She, as is typical for someone suffering with a Major Depressive Episode, struggled with feelings of excessive or inappropriate guilt, worthlessness and low self-esteem, especially as her ability to function continued to deteriorate.

When this occurs it is extremely debilitating, as it becomes part of the downward spiral of depression. The worse one feels, the more immobilized she becomes, which in turn makes her feel even worse, and so on. People in the midst of a Major Depressive Episode lose perspective of a reasonable sense of responsibility and accountability and get stuck in unreasonable self blame. In severe cases, this may reach delusional proportions.[113]

Psychomotor Changes

When the fatigue of depression sets in, people may also experience psychomotor retardation. Psychomotor issues address the level of bodily activity including speech (speed, volume, content and enthusiasm), bodily movements, the speed of thinking and responsiveness. When there is psychomotor retardation, activity is slowed down to such abnormal levels that it is easily observed by others. For example, they may speak so softly you can barely hear them or they may appear to be moving in slow motion, requiring a great effort to accomplish a simple task. Lifting a spoon may look like one is lifting a brick.

Conversely, Major Depressive Episode may be characterized by psychomotor agitation. In the case of psychomotor agitation, there may be nervousness in the body movements such as picking, pulling, pacing or fidgeting. You may notice in these individuals that they are practically yelling when speaking or speaking so fast you find it nearly impossible to understand them. They will appear to be antsy—constantly moving and shifting.

Cognitive Impacts

Those with Major Depressive Episode are also impaired in the cognitive realm. Concentration, memory, thinking and decision-making may all suffer. Such depressed individuals complain of loss of memory and/or of being easily distracted. These impairments are not sporadic or momentary. They are very different from the perimenopausal lapses that may cause you to pour orange juice in your coffee instead of cream. This type of memory loss, a symptom of depression, occurs on a continual, regular, daily basis. This can be very frightening since most people do not understand that these sorts of cognitive challenges are symptoms of depression. It is not uncommon for depressed individuals to self-diagnose attention deficit disorders or even dementia when the cognitive effects of this type of depression are extreme. Fortunately, when the depressive episode is resolved, these cognitive impairments disappear.

Suicidal Thoughts

The most serious concern for those suffering from a Major Depressive Episode is the risk of suicide. When there is excessive rumination about killing oneself or dying, a suicide attempt may be carried out. Often the suicidal ideation is an extension of feelings of worthlessness, but it can also be a result of the hopelessness of existing in such a devastating emotional state, one that appears to have no solution or happy ending.

When Suzanne reached this level of hopelessness, it became apparent to those around her that her depression was serious. Obviously, this is an extremely dangerous aspect of Major Depressive Episode. Major depression, which strikes women twice as frequently as men,[114] can cause more disability and impairments in a woman's physical and social functioning than many serious medical conditions. One must always take seriously the condition of a depressed loved one who is experiencing utter hopelessness.

Major Depressive Disorder

Major Depressive Disorder (MDD) is diagnosed when there have been one or more occurrences of Major Depressive Episode in an individual. The course of MDD can be very variable. Some individuals may have isolated episodes of depression separated by long periods of time with complete remission of symptoms. Others may have episodes that cluster more frequently. A serious concern for anyone suffering with MDD is the risk of suicide. As many as 15 percent of those diagnosed with MDD die as a result of suicide. Those over the age of fifty-five with this disorder are four times as likely to die.

MDD is a very serious type of depression and needs to be addressed as such.[115] Not only is the risk of death due to suicide very high, it has the potential to disrupt healthy functioning, more severely than serious medical diseases. The severe symptoms of MDD may result in disability, inability to earn an income, lack of ability to care for oneself or one's family, an inability to maintain social connections and the loss of hope and desire to get well. Each of these symptoms has the potential to exacerbate the others and to make recovery from MDD even harder. Most individuals with MDD require a concerned friend or relative to initiate the process to get help.

MDD, similar to Major Depressive Episode, is twice as prevalent in females, both adolescent and adult, than in males of the same age category. It has been reported in community based research that up to 25 percent of women have a lifetime risk for developing MDD while men have a risk of up to 12 percent. This means that one in four women are at risk for succumbing to this type of depression. This is a huge number. Interestingly, prior to puberty the prevalence of developing this disorder is the same in males and females. This may suggest the role of hormones in the etiology of depression in females.

The profound hormonal shifts in perimenopause can certainly generate the conditions in which one who is predisposed to MDD may succumb. Certain medical conditions, the presence of extreme psychosocial stressors and a family history of depression are also implicated in contributing to the onset of such depression. Family history is such a strong predictor that someone who has a first degree relative with MDD, will have a one and one half to a three times greater likelihood of developing the same disorder.

Dysthymic Disorder

Dysthymic Disorder can best be described as a lighter depression than MDD but is continuous and lasts much longer. In order to be diagnosed with Dysthymic Disorder, one needs to be in a depressed mood most of the time for a period of at least two years. People with Dysthymic Disorder feel sad or "blue." They will experience changes in their appetite that can induce either overeating or under-eating. Similar to other types of depression, those suffering with Dysthymic Disorder will have trouble sleeping, fatigue, trouble concentrating, low self-esteem, feelings of hopelessness, difficulty making decisions and self-deprecating thoughts and statements. Unfortunately, Dysthymic Disorder is a risk factor for MDD; 10 percent of those diagnosed with Dysthymic Disorder later go on to have a Major Depressive Episode.[116]

Adjustment Disorder with Depressed Mood

An Adjustment Disorder would be diagnosed in a symptomatic individual who has been exposed to a specific psychosocial stressor within the prior three months. There are emotional or behavioral symptoms that indicate a level of distress that is disproportionate to what would typically occur in such a situation. There may also be a serious disruption in social, occupational or academic functioning.[117]

This was the case with Anne. After an incident in which Anne got into minor trouble with the law, she found herself so distraught she was unable to work or take care of herself. She was forced to move back home with her parents for several months until she was able to cope again. After this recovery period, Anne was back to fully functioning with appropriate mood and affect with no further difficulty.

An Adjustment Disorder is short-lived, lasting a maximum of six months after exposure to the stressor. If the stressor is lasting, continuous or there are a series of stressors, the Adjustment Disorder may last longer than six months. Adjustment Disorder with Depressed Mood is diagnosed when the manifestations of symptoms are sadness in nature. Tearfulness, feelings of hopelessness, and sadness are the dominant feelings in response to the stressor. Although the depth of depressed feelings is not as deep as in some of the other Depressive Disorders, Adjustment Disorder with Depressed Mood is associated with an increased risk of suicidal behaviors, both attempts and completed suicides. Both women and men are equally susceptible to developing Adjustment Disorders, which sets it apart from some of the other depressive disorders. This suggests that hormones do not influence the development of this condition, making it less of a risk in perimenopause than other types of depression.

Mood Disorder Due to a General Medical Condition

Mood Disorder Due to a General Medical Condition encompasses a disturbance in mood that may be expansive, elevated or irritable, as in Bipolar Disorders, or depressed with diminished pleasure in life as in the Depressive Disorders. I will limit this section to the *Mood Disorder Due to a General Medical Condition with Depressive Features.*

What differentiates Mood Disorder Due to a General Medical Condition from the other Mood Disorders is that in this disorder a general, identifiable medical condition is the direct cause of the disturbance in mood.[118] If the medical condition is resolved, the mood disorder is resolved.

Symptoms of Mood Disorder Due to a General Medical Condition are feelings of sadness, hopelessness, or diminished interest in life as in the other mood disorders, but they may vary in intensity depending on the type of medical condition. There may be sleep disturbances, appetite changes and cognitive difficulties also similar to the other Depressive Disorders, again varying in accordance to the physiological condition. *Mood Disorder Due to a General Medical Condition With Depressive Features* will also present with feelings of worthlessness, fatigue and guilt along with suicidal ideation and/or completed suicides as we have seen in the other types of depression. Because this type of depression is directly linked to a medical condition, the likelihood of males and females developing this disorder is similar, as is the case with Adjustment Disorder with Depressed Mood.

One example of a Mood Disorder Due to a General Medical Condition would be thyroid disorders. We will learn in Chapter 26 how thyroid disorders, specifically hypothyroidism, can create symptoms of depression. The slowed metabolism, a result of hypothyroidism, causes sleep disturbances, lethargy, fatigue, foggy thinking and depression. When this continues over time, the hypothyroid individual begins to feel hopeless and despondent. As her productivity wanes, relationships are challenged and life becomes more and more difficult, inviting depression to set in. In such an individual, treating the hypothyroidism may resolve the depression but there may also be some residual depressive symptomotology. The hypothyroidism would require treatment first and then the individual would need to be treated for any remaining depression.

The case is similarly made for depression that results from perimenopause, with one exception. Perimenopause, similar to hypothyroidism, is a condition ruled by a significant change in hormone levels. One major difference between hypothyroidism and perimenopause is that hypothyroidism is an abnormal medical state that warrants correcting for the health of the individual. Perimenopause is a normal condition that does not necessarily warrant correcting unless there are difficult and complicating symptoms that interfere with happy and healthy living.

Depending on the physiology in a particular woman, the depressive symptoms a perimenopausal woman is experiencing may indicate the presence of one of the Depressive Disorders or a Mood Disorder Due to a

General Medical Condition. An experienced psychologist or psychiatrist would be able to make that distinction after taking her history and examining her symptoms. When depression is a result of the general medical condition of perimenopause, the perimenopausal irregularity should be treated in order to facilitate treatment of the depression. This does not imply that the perimenopause must be treated in order to treat the depression, but the implications of perimenopausal symptoms must be understood and considered for any treatment plan.

An example of this complication is that perimenopause induced depression tends to be cyclical or variable as the estrogen levels shift radically. To the uninformed observer, the depression may more closely resemble Bipolar Disorder, which is characterized by extreme mood fluctuations. A moody perimenopausal woman is not necessarily bipolar-certainly not simply due to erratic hormones. The nature of the shifting hormones of perimenopause tells a very different story. The fluctuating moods are simply due to the fluctuating hormones. Once the hormones are stabilized, the moods stabilize. This would not be the case if a woman was truly bipolar. Treatment options for perimenopause will be reviewed later in Chapter 24, but it is important to understand the origination of the depression, as well as the type of depression in order to treat it effectively and responsibly.

Chapter Seventeen

Who Is at Risk for Depression?

Biological Factors

*I*n the general population, depression, which includes, but is not limited to the range of Depressive Disorders described above, is estimated to occur in as many as 33 percent of individuals. Depressive Disorders affect females far more frequently than males. Not surprisingly, depressive symptoms are most frequent in times of dramatic hormonal change, the periods of menarche, perimenopause and postpartum.[119, 120] The hormonal changes of menstrual cycling impact the neuromodulators (the brain chemicals involved in mood disorders) such as serotonin, creating the connection between female hormonal changes and depression.[121]

This hormonal cycling affects a majority of women through its actions on neuromodulators which creates a vulnerability to psychosocial, sociocultural, environmental and psychological impingements. Studies have indicated that as many as 75 percent of women experience PMS to some degree.[122] Since there is a high correlation between women who suffer from PMS and postpartum depression and with those who later are perimenopausal and suffer from affective symptoms,[123] it becomes clear that those who are vulnerable, are vulnerable throughout all of their reproductive years. The correlation is so strong between depression in PMS and perimenopause that depression in PMS can be a predictor for depression in perimenopause.[124]

Fluctuating estradiol, one of the estrogens, has been identified as a strong risk factor in the onset of depression during times of hormonal change.[125] In perimenopause when estradiol fluctuates widely we see very high rates of depression.[126, 127, 128] In understanding that estrogen is instrumental in reducing the breakdown of serotonin and has a positive effect on intraneural transport of serotonin, we learn that stable levels of estrogen will have a mood enhancing effect.

Both of these mechanisms make more serotonin available, which improves mood and reduces depression.[129] The previous chapter allowed us to see how the various depressive symptoms may worsen one another and also how they are impacted by sleep disruption, appetite irregularities, low energy levels, decreased cognitive abilities and poor concentration. Now we see how the initially vacillating and later falling levels of estrogen increase the risk of, and may even be the direct cause of developing depression.

In one study as many as 45 percent of perimenopausal women were diagnosed as clinically depressed. Thirty five percent of the women were experiencing clinical depression for the first time.[130] Other researchers have found that the risk of depression triples as women proceed through perimenopause.[131] Still other research has shown that women with no prior history of depression were four times as likely to exhibit some signs of depression during perimenopause, and over twice as likely to suffer from clinical depression.[132]

This is also true of MDD (Major Depressive Disorder). The frequency of MDD is higher in the perimenopausal period, compared to premenopause and postmenopause, even if there has been no history of MDD in the individual.[133] When there is a positive premenopausal history of MDD in an individual, that then becomes a very strong predictor for another occurrence of such depression during perimenopause.[134, 135]

One study found that 83 percent of clinically depressed perimenopausal women had suffered from depression at a prior time.[136]

Another risk factor for depression in perimenopause is family history of depression. Women who have a family history of depression are much more vulnerable to suffering from a major depression when they are perimenopausal than those women without a family history of depression, especially when they experience more serious and stressful life events,[137] such as health related issues, everyday stressors, stresses due to lack of social support or significant changes in family life.

What all of this means, is that there is a high percentage of women that suffer from depressive symptoms and from more serious clinical depression during perimenopause. It is understood that the hormonal fluctuations of perimenopause may lower the threshold for susceptibility to depression especially when there are stressful challenges happening in the woman's life in addition to the direct stresses of perimenopause.

The risk of developing depression increases further when a woman has a positive personal history with depression and/or a family history of depression. Those women with a positive history for depression should be more aware of their susceptibility to suffering depressive symptoms when they enter perimenopause. The encouraging side to this is that most problems with depression exist three to four years before the completion of menstruation. Once menses have ceased, the prevalence of Depressive Disorders drops off.[138]

Vasomotor Factors

When Shirley passed the halfway point of perimenopause she began experiencing severe vasomotor symptoms. Like clockwork, every hour, day and night the heat crept up her spine and exploded in a drenching sweat from her waist all the way up into her scalp. Because of the severity of her vasomotor symptoms, Shirley was at higher risk for developing depression during perimenopause.[139] Recent research[140] has indicated that women who have challenging vasomotor symptoms have an increased risk for depression. This risk can be as much as a six-fold increase for suffering from an episode of depression.[141]

Vasomotor symptoms include flushes, commonly referred to as "hot flashes" and night sweats. Falling estrogen levels and ovarian failure during perimenopause create a dysregulation in the thermoregulatory centers in the brain that are expressed as hot flashes. Nocturnal hot flashes, also referred to as night sweats, can produce extreme amounts of perspiration and sweating. Women, like Shirley, report awakening in a state of mild to extreme wetness, sometimes to the extent of requiring a clothing or bedding change in the middle of the night. Shirley kept a towel and a spare pair of pajamas next to her bed so she could dry off and change.

Vasomotor symptoms, in the extreme, create significant disruptions in sleep, leading to exhaustion and difficulty in daily functioning. This domino effect becomes a tangled web in which it becomes difficult to tease apart what part of the depressive symptoms is due to the hormonal changes of perimenopause and what part is due to the effects of severe sleep disruption and deprivation.

While we know that female hormonal changes are influential in creating affective disorders, the relationship is not fully understood. There are multiple hypotheses being researched to better understand this process. What is known is that the ovarian hormones have a complex interaction with the central nervous system. These hormones directly affect many of the activities of neuromodulators (the brain chemicals involved in mood disorders) by influencing their creation, release, absorption, activation/inactivation and how they are received by receptors.[142, 143]

Women with premenstrual dysphoric disorder (PMDD), a severe cousin to PMS, have been found to have altered serotonin (a neurotransmitter) function similar to that found in affective disorders.[144] Hence, PMDD is responsive to treatment with SSRIs, as is depression.[145] Thankfully, new research is underway to gain a more complete understanding as to how all of these systems interact in the woman's body. We, in the psychological community, look forward to a time when women no longer feel misunderstood or patronized because they experience changes in their moods or sense of wellbeing as they travel through life hormonally and emotionally.

As we have seen with anxiety, the many physiological changes taking place in the body during perimenopause, primarily initiated by hormonal changes, create psychological effects. Also, as in the case of developing anxiety, there are many life events that contribute to feelings of depression at this time. When depression sets in, depending on its severity, it can become extremely debilitating. In its most severe forms it will incapacitate the individual while having a deleterious effect on all of those around.

Psychosocial Factors

In our culture the passage through perimenopause often coincides with some enormous life challenges. The psychosocial difficulties that women in their forties and fifties may face are: coping with aging parents, pubescent children, preparing for retirement or children's college and the changing emotional dynamic with peers as women and their families mature. These difficulties, as we have learned, may create symptoms of anxiety but they are equally likely to create symptoms of depression. For women who are mothers, one of the most difficult of these challenges is the "'empty nest syndrome." The empty nest occurs when the youngest child leaves home. The "empty nest syndrome" refers to the adjustments a mother must make emotionally, psychologically and practically when her stage of active parenting comes to an end.

Although some theorists believe that depression associated with the empty nest syndrome is limited to those women who are excessively engaged with their children,[146] I have found this not to be the case. In my clinical practice I have seen women who have appropriate, healthy engagement with their children, have extensive friendship networks and have pursued their own interests, whether in careers or hobbies, suffer significantly when their nests initially become empty. Mood disorders are not infrequently the outcome.

The combination of the hormonal shifts with the overwhelming impact of such a huge change in lifestyle and daily functioning is a lot for a woman to handle. The majority of women who are susceptible to being overcome at this juncture suffer from *Adjustment Disorder with Depressed Mood* as opposed to the more serious Depressive Disorders. I described earlier how this is a relatively short-lived disorder, lasting less than six months. It is a reaction to a defined situation that creates the shift in mood and coping ability. Women need some time to adapt to this dramatic shift in their responsibilities, identities and feelings.

Women who have raised children have typically spent over twenty-five years bringing all of their children from birth to emancipation. Depending on the spacing of the children, this time frame can be even longer. After so many years of viewing oneself as "Johnny's mother" or "Suzie's mom," it is an arduous task to suddenly shift perspective and view oneself differently. Women struggle with what their value is, now that there are no children at home to care for. The smallest things become a reminder of this difference, such as taking out that extra dinner plate when setting the table. How many times a day does a mother look at the clock, thinking 'Dan will be home any minute', only to realize Dan will not be home until Thanksgiving break. These women begin to worry how they will fill their time. The entire rhythm of each day, each week changes. Can they redefine themselves now that their children are on their own? How do they go about doing so? All of the things they always wanted to have time to do suddenly do not seem quite so appealing. How does one begin to think of herself as an "I" when for the last twenty-five years she has always thought of herself as a "we"?

Nancy's Nest

Nancy is a forty eight year old mother of two. She is aware that she has been perimenopausal for a couple of years. More recently, her period has become very irregular. This happened to coincide with her youngest child leaving for college. Nancy had always been a very involved mother. She considered herself close to her two sons but admitted that in many ways the boys were closer to their father. Regardless, she was involved in their sports' activities and kept abreast of their social and academic endeavors.

Nancy showed appropriate involvement and concern for her children although she did tend to get caught up in worrying about them at times. Nancy had always worked part time in a family run business. She was close with her parents and her siblings and had a few close friends. Her marriage was healthy and satisfying.

When Nancy's older son left for college it was very difficult for her. Her older child was always the more independent of the two; she was reasonably confident he would fare well, and he did.

After two years, her younger son left for college, leaving her with an empty nest. This was when Nancy faced a much greater challenge. The fabric of her daily life was so notably changed that Nancy had a great deal of trouble adjusting. She began to feel more and more uncomfortable.

Initially, Nancy had some trouble sleeping. She attributed this to worrying about some issues her son was having at school, but she was also having some very intense night sweats. She began to feel "down" a lot of the time. She was losing her energy and her pep. Simultaneously, she began gaining weight. Daily chores became more and more difficult to begin and to complete. Nancy was afraid to share her struggle with her friends for fear they would think she was "losing it." She cut down on her work schedule but found that she had nothing interesting or enticing to fill the time with. Nancy shared her feelings with her husband. He tried to be supportive, but this was not the Nancy he knew. He found it very hard to find words or actions that would help her to feel better.

After about five months, Nancy began to feel better. Although the night sweats continued, Nancy's sleep difficulties were beginning to ease. She started feeling more energetic in her daily life and returned to her prior level of activity and involvement. By this time, Nancy was reaching out to others, to both professionals

*and friends, in an effort to understand what was happening and
what others were experiencing.*

*She found a great deal of comfort in realizing that her symp-
toms and her feelings were part of an integrated system of hormonal and psychosocial changes that were happening to her at
that time. Interestingly, four months after her younger son left for
college, Nancy began skipping periods. The easing of her emotional symptoms coincided with her transition from perimenopause
into menopause, all facilitated by her reaching out for help and
understanding. This transition also facilitated her adjustment to
her empty nest. Had she not gained the support and the understanding, she may possibly have deteriorated into a more serious
and prolonged struggle with depression.*

Psychodynamic Issues

A notable challenge that married women face at this juncture of their
lives is the re-negotiation of the marital relationship with their husbands.
When a couple initially brings children into their union, the relationship
shifts from one of friends and lovers to coparents of their mutual children. This relationship shift undergoes a reversal when the children grow
up and leave the home. Even the couples that are extremely successful
at maintaining their relationship as friends and lovers throughout the
childrearing years undergo a process of reacquainting themselves with
each other in that role once the children have left the home. More typically, husband and wife have lost some degree of relating to one another
and must undergo a process of familiarizing themselves with each other
in a whole new emotional environment. This additional challenge can
initially leave a woman feeling lost, alone and disconnected from her
husband.

For a mother, not having the children to focus on leaves her without the diversion that has kept her busy for the many preceding years.
Even when a woman has a satisfying career or outside interests, the impact of children leaving home is typically more significant for mothers

than for fathers. Mothers tend to be more involved in their parental roles throughout the day than are fathers. This is partially because men are more inclined to compartmentalize the different sectors of their lives. At work, they are focused on work. When they are home, they are focused on home and the children.

With women, the lines are much more blurred. At work their attention will be divided between work responsibilities and the children. A woman might be in the midst of an important assignment and have the thought pass through her mind that her daughter's biology test just started. She is less likely to keep work and home separate the way her husband does. This makes the impact of adjusting to these changes much more difficult for women.

How easily husband and wife transition back into being a couple will be influenced by how well a woman's partner is able to relate to these difficulties and show support for her feelings and needs. It is not uncommon for the couple to find the journey back to each other to be a bit bumpy and even turbulent. This additional psychosocial and psychodynamic complication may increase a perimenopausal woman's susceptibility to depression.

Relationship issues can be an even bigger risk factor for the onset of depression in perimenopausal women who are divorced or widowed. Many single women decide to postpone any serious consideration of a couple's relationship while they are raising their children. Single women may confront, for the first time in many years, the prospect of returning to dating or engaging in a serious relationship.

The hurdles of reacquainting herself with her femininity and sexuality with a new partner have unique challenges for the single perimenopausal woman. While these insecurities also affect women who are not single, they are more difficult for those who are. The ways in which a woman experiences and perceives herself sexually is changing as her hormonal changes make their imprint. Her libido is not as reliable as it was in her premenopausal years. The changes in her body, in terms of weight gain, and skin changes, including the appearance of lines and wrinkles, loss of elasticity or age spots may make a women self-conscious when considering dating.

Along with her struggles regarding her self-image, the single peri-menopausal woman's declining energy levels may make dating seem overwhelming. The plans she may have held for the eventuality of her children leaving home are not shaping up the way she had imagined. When her children finally do leave the home, she will certainly feel the loss quite acutely. Depending on the support systems such a woman has in place, she will be more or less likely to struggle with depression.

Single women who have developed interests outside of the home and their children will experience an easier transition when their nests empty out. Friends, whether male or female, that either have empty nests or are going through it with them will help with the transition and perhaps reduce the risk of succumbing to depression. The more engaged women are with jobs, volunteer and social activities, the less likely they will be completely lost when their last child leaves home.

A supportive family system is also a tremendous help. Women who have isolated themselves from other people and activities and made their entire existence revolve around their children are the ones most at risk for developing depressive symptoms when faced with the dual challenge of perimenopause and the empty nest. This risk is even greater when there are financial difficulties.[147]

Three Strikes for Angela

Angela, at 51, was suffering from a Major Depressive Episode. She had been divorced for two years. The breakup of her marriage had been her ex-husband's choice. Although the marriage was not healthy, Angela had been willing to "stick it out," at least until the children left home. Now Angela was divorced, her oldest child was in college; her youngest was just two years behind. Angela began to have some emotional difficulties adjusting to the knowledge that in only two years she would have no one left at home.

Angela had never worked since having her children. She had been very happy to stay home, raise the children and take care of the house and family. Unfortunately, Angela had had little time or energy to develop interests of her own. Her time had been spent enjoying the activities of her children, watching them perform and making the home welcoming to their friends. Over the years, she had become a reflection of everyone else's needs and had quite lost herself in the process.

When Angela began experiencing symptoms of depression, she was also at the peak of her perimenopause. She had severe insomnia during the night, but slept often during the day. She felt despondent much of the time; her energy was almost nil and everything she had to do took an enormous effort. She lost nearly 25 pounds and found herself withdrawing more and more from friends and family. She swore she would never be able to date again.

Angela had a triple blow: divorce, perimenopause and empty nest all happening within a short period of time. Angela began to understand through her work in therapy that her healing would come about in rebuilding her own life. By the time her youngest left for college, she had begun a career, pursuing an interest she had pushed aside for many years while raising her children.

She became active in her church, which gave her access to new friends. Angela discovered there were many interesting church activities for which she became a frequent volunteer. She took a step back from her concern with her children, which allowed more time and energy to focus on herself. Eventually, Angela began planning to sell her house in order to free herself financially and practically from the burdens of taking care of a house alone. Her depression began to lift, she completed perimenopause and sailed smoothly into menopause. To finish her story, Angela the woman who had sworn off dating embarked on a serious flirtation with a charming man with whom she was acquainted.

Chapter Eighteen
The Bottom Line

$\mathscr{A}$s estrogen levels begin to drop, women have a higher risk for suffering from depression. The risk exists whether or not women have or do not have personal or family histories of depression. The risk exists regardless of how vastly their menstrual cycles shift or how many vasomotor challenges they may have. The perimenopausal woman is more likely to suffer from depression whether or not her sleep is mildly or grossly affected, whether she takes care of aging parents or has children leaving the nest. All of these factors influence how great or small the risk and how severe or mild the symptoms, but the risk is still ever present. What exactly is going on?

More of the recent research is looking toward the connection between estrogen and the neurotransmitter, serotonin, for the etiology of depression during perimenopause.[148] The exact interaction of these two substances in the body is far from being understood but research continues to try to get to the bottom of it. Whenever we look at changes in neurotransmitter levels, we are faced with the age-old chicken-and-egg question. Do outside psychological events cause an alteration of neurotransmitter levels or do the changing levels of neurotransmitters (due to any physiological event) cause the psychological issues. The answer is not definitive but there is reason to believe the effect is mutual; psychological distress causes changes in neurotransmitter levels, and physiological events that change neurotransmitter levels will result in psychological symptoms. Of course, we do know that the more challenges a woman has, in terms of the biological, psychosocial, psychodynamic and vasomotor issues, the greater the risk of onset of depression and the more serious the depression is likely to be. The following case describes a dream Rachel had. It is a wonderful example of the many issues women are struggling with at this stage of their lives and how they come together to alter their moods.

Letting Go of Fertility

Rachel had been in perimenopause for a couple of years. She had always considered herself a very sensitive and nurturing woman. She was an extremely devoted mother and fostered close, loving relationships with her children and husband.

Rachel had always had a particularly difficult time with hormonal changes, and perimenopause was no exception. She struggled with depression from early on in her perimenopausal transition. One morning, Rachel awoke, extremely distressed after having a disturbing dream. She dreamt that she had had a third child, a daughter, and was determined not to make any mistakes as she might have made with her first two children.

In the dream she was unable to carry this child in pregnancy, but had to have a surrogate. Because she had not been pregnant she was unable to nurse the baby. She was quite frustrated and upset as she watched others bottle-feed her baby, while knowing the surrogate had an ample supply of breast milk to give her tiny daughter and she had none. The overriding feeling Rachel had in this dream was that this newborn child was hers, but not hers. It was hers genetically, but another had carried it, birthed it and was now feeding it. Upon awakening, Rachel felt very agitated and depressed.

Analysis of this dream with Rachel highlighted a number of critical events that Rachel was struggling with in her life. One of the themes that jumps right out, is the ending of Rachel's reproductive ability. One can see that her inability to produce a child on her own is a function of the transition perimenopause brings.

She shows us her unconscious reconciliation of this in her dream as she explored bringing an infant into her world in which she was a step removed. She was having a baby that was not quite her own, but felt as if it was somewhat hers. This was, for Rachel, a symbol for anticipating the next "maternal" stage of life; becoming a grandmother. Rachel was leaving behind her own childbearing years as her children got older and were moving into the adult phase of their own lives...but she was simultaneously moving closer to her children becoming parents.

A second theme that emerges in the dream is that of Rachel's recent separation from her youngest child, her daughter. Rachel's daughter had left for her first year at college a short time earlier. Rachel's close relationship with her daughter allowed for a lot of daily involvement and help on Rachel's part with her daughter's college preparation. We can see the conflicted feelings in Rachel's unconscious mind represented in the dream of her wanting to nurture and feed the infant with her own body, but having to allow someone else to take over. Here we can see quite clearly the struggle Rachel is having with her empty nest, and progressing through her youngest child's growth from dependence to independence.

Rachel's dream was a brilliant representation of how so many factors come together to challenge a woman's sense of wellbeing at this time of her life. The hormonal changes of perimenopause, the empty nest, the emancipation of children, the doubts about how well she parented her children now that her job was done (represented by her not wanting to repeat prior mistakes), the end of the child-bearing years and the redefining of oneself as other than mom are all contributors to emotional difficulties women face. It is no wonder that Rachel awoke depressed after having all of this come together in one dream!

In the end, our chicken-and egg-dilemma, or the means by which serotonin and estrogen interact is secondary to the understanding that women are very susceptible to depression at this time of their lives, perhaps more susceptible than at any other time. This is primarily because of all of the hormonal and other major life events that come together. They encounter an onslaught of difficult issues in a relatively short period of time when physiologically they are compromised by fluctuating hormones. In cases of severe depression, women suffer greatly. By disentangling the issues and allowing women and their loved ones to make sense of the confusion, we can support them in their struggle through this challenging time.

Chapter Nineteen

The Face of Depression

Too often the term "depression" is over used in common language. People will talk about being depressed when they are simply sad or feeling down. A state of clinical depression involves the symptomotology described previously. The exact type of depression is diagnosed according to which symptoms a person has, and how severe and lasting they are. The frequency with which people speak incorrectly of being depressed can contribute to neglecting those who are truly clinically depressed. This may lead to a situation in which many women are depressed without knowing it or getting the proper interventions.

The internal and external experiences of depression may be different. The internal experience is typically one of fatigue, sadness and futility or of feeling overwhelmed. A depressed woman may feel somewhat tired, listless or disinterested. If she is accustomed to experiencing PMS, she may be familiar with feeling downturns in her mood periodically. As depression evolves, her energy levels will drop significantly. The events and activities that once gave her pleasure will offer little or no enjoyment.

A depressed woman may find herself drifting back into bed once the family has left and started their day. She knows the laundry basket is overflowing with dirty clothes and she should get up to wash them. She knows the dishes need to be done and the house needs tidying. She has a list of calls to make and errands to run but all she can feel is hopelessness and fatigue. Before she knows it, the day has passed and she has done nothing. She considers this a marginal success; this was the first time in a week that she managed to get showered and dressed. Maybe, she prays, she will be able to make dinner for her family tonight instead of ordering in again.

The external expression of depression is often misinterpreted to be laziness or lack of caring. Her family will notice the changes in her habits and behavior. To those around her, she may just appear to be "under the weather." They see her productivity decreasing. When questioned, the depressed woman will likely be unable to give much of an answer. A simple question or request reduces her to tears. Every day she awakens with promises to herself that she will do better. She finds herself crying in the shower every morning as she tries to start each day. The depression is just too powerful. As lost days accumulate, she will begin to feel more and more dejected, more remorse, and more shame. She may find herself explaining to her family that she was tired, while trying to figure out for herself what is wrong and why she cannot pull herself out of this. She does not know herself anymore. She is a stranger to the image that looks back at her in the mirror.

While in the grips of depression, a woman will find it challenging to maintain her concentration. This will be exacerbated if she is also peri-menopausal. She finds herself easily confused and forgetful. Her children may be frustrated with the things she has forgotten to do. The permission slip that needed to be signed is nowhere to be found. She never did place that phone call to the plumber. The incident described to her, in exquisite detail only the day before is gone from her memory. Try as she may, she just cannot bring it back.

To her family members, these behaviors in their wife/mother are very frightening. Their perception of her is as withdrawn, detached, uninvolved and perhaps uncaring. The helplessness so characteristic of the depressed woman may begin to seep into the other family members. When depression is significant and prolonged, as in MDD, the family and friends become lost and confused. The severely depressed individual is unreachable. She does not know what can help her or cheer her. What she may desire most is to be left alone, to sleep and to be allowed to disengage from everyone and everything. She may be aware of how frightening and unhealthy her behavior is for her family but she is helpless to change it. This awareness will create in her a deepening sense of worthlessness. The typical healthy woman is such a pivotal figure in the functioning of her family, that when depression sets in, it is a tremendously violent, albeit silent upheaval.

Chapter Twenty
Treatment for Depression

*T*he two most common and successful treatments for depression are different types of psychotherapy and medication-based treatment using antidepressants. It is important to understand what type of depression one is dealing with in order to best assess the treatment modality for that individual. It has been shown that there is no difference in the efficacy of either psychotherapy or medication-based treatment when treating mild to moderate depression. In severely and chronically depressed individuals, a combination of therapy and medication offers the most positive results.[149] Antidepressant treatment, alone, is effective in only 65 to 70 percent of depressed individuals.

Clearly, when depression is the result of a medical condition, the depression must be treated in conjunction with the medical condition. For example, as we will see in Chapter 26, hypothyroidism is a medical condition that often causes depressive symptoms. If a woman is depressed and hypothyroid, psychotherapy will only provide partial relief of her depressive symptoms until her thyroid condition is treated. By the same token, if a woman is depressed because she is perimenopausal, the treatment must address the hormonal issues in order to effectively treat the depression.

If the depression is not a result of perimenopause but coincides with it, each issue must be addressed in order for the woman to feel her best. This does not imply that the depression should not be treated if the physiological cause is not treated.

There are many women in perimenopause who choose not to treat their hormonal issues. They would still benefit from antidepressant medication and psychotherapy. However, it would be advantageous for these women to understand the physiological process that is influencing their mood. They would experience better results from the treatment they are getting if they grasp the impact of the hormones and how, why and when various hormonal changes will affect their depression. This is why it is so beneficial for women to be educated about their bodily processes and for the medical and psychological communities to work together when an individual presents with integrated and entangled physiological and psychological issues.

When depression is not severe, therapy alone may be a successful treatment course. It also can be successful in some cases of severe depression. Different types of therapy, whether individual, marital or family therapy have shown success in preventing the reoccurrence of major depression in patients. Support groups are another alternative for receiving emotional support when depressed. Having others with whom you can share experiences and gain empathy is very uplifting for the depressed individual. Giving support can be as beneficial as receiving support because it allows the depressed individual to feel empowered, diminishing her feelings of helplessness.

In cases where depression is profound, medication is usually indicated in addition to psychotherapy. Interestingly, there is a gender difference regarding responsivity to different antidepressant medications. Men respond better to tricyclic antidepressants while premenopausal women respond better to selective serotonin reuptake inhibitors (SSRIs). Once women are postmenopausal, this difference disappears, suggesting there are gender differences in the levels of serotonin in the central nervous system of premenopausal women and men.[150]

SSRIs have some advantages over tricyclic antidepressants. The SSRIs have very few and very mild side effects and they have no risk for lethal overdose.[151] When a profoundly depressed individual is initially treated with any type of antidepressant medication, the risk of suicide increases for a short period of time and should be monitored closely. This would be a time to increase the support and attention to a depressed loved one.

There are other alternative treatments for depression that show many beneficial effects. These treatments include hormonal treatments, eastern therapies such as acupuncture, yoga and meditation, dietary improvements, exercise and taking supplements. These will be reviewed in more detail in Chapter 24 when all of the challenges of perimenopause will be integrated with various treatment solutions.

Chapter Twenty-one

Perimenopausal Women
with Prior Emotional Issues

here are some women for whom perimenopause may exacerbate psychological problems with which they have already
been struggling. This applies to problems that may or may not have been
professionally diagnosed. Occasionally women may have been mildly
or unobtrusively symptomatic. They may have thought of themselves
as "quirky" or "a little bit rigid." In this chapter we will see how the
challenges of perimenopause can bring such problems into the realm of
full-fledged psychological disorders. Because the effects of the changing hormones are so pervasive throughout the body, nearly every bodily
function or emotional weakness may become vulnerable with the onset
of perimenopause. There are a few categories of psychological distress
that frequently worsen as perimenopause gets underway.

Substance Abuse

Substance abuse falls into three main categories: alcohol abuse, prescription medication abuse and non-prescription substance abuse. In my

practice I have seen an increase in abuse in all three categories in peri-menopausal women. As the disturbances of perimenopause impact mind and body, women who previously have had unhealthy methods of cop-ing, frequently find even more dysfunctional ways to cope. They tend to get into trouble when they adopt a mindset of "one more drink or an extra Xanax will help me feel calmer." When this becomes habitual, a woman may find herself with a substance abuse problem.

The woman who is more likely to fall into this sort of difficulty will have maladaptive coping strategies. She may cope via avoidance. She would be a type of person who avoids facing the obvious changes hap-pening within her body or in her life. She may be in denial that she is in perimenopause. She may not want to acknowledge how distressing life changes may be- for example that her youngest child has moved out or she is affected by changing emotional dynamics with her partner. Rather than delve into an emotional, hormonal or physical problem and sort through it, she finds an escape in substances or by self-medicating. She is more likely to reach for that bottle of wine or jar of pills than talk with a trusted friend or therapist.

Historically, this avoidant woman has avoided feeling life's pain by using drugs or medication. In past episodes of difficulty she may have been able to cope by using a reasonable, safe amount of her preferred substance, but now things begin to change. With the added strain of per-imenopausal hormonal changes, the substance dependent woman may find herself using more, even much more, of her preferred vice.

In other cases the presence of depression in perimenopause may be the catalyst, provoking a woman to search for chemical relief. As we have already learned, the hormonal changes in perimenopause frequently in-crease anxiety tremendously, especially when in Stages II and III, Emo-tional Disruption and Turbulence, respectively. It is this overwhelming anxiety that may promote a choice to utilize a substance in order to calm down or cope.

Sometimes it is the extreme sleep disruption that may push a woman in an unhealthy direction. This can start when she begins using a drink or a sedative to help her sleep. The sleep deprived or depressed woman may overdose on caffeine or take a stimulant to function during the day, creating a dangerous cycle of substance dependence. This woman may have flirted with addictive behavior throughout her life, but now slides right down that slippery slope into clinical substance abuse. Whether her substance of choice is alcohol, a sedative, marijuana, stimulants or any combination of these, she is now in need of professional help and support.

Janie's Addiction

Janie is a good example of a wonderful woman who fell into such a pattern. Janie went through surgical menopause, menopause following a hysterectomy. Janie was always prone to anxiety and had frequently obtained prescriptions for a sedative from her doctor to manage the more difficult times. When her hormonal state began to shift dramatically following her surgery, Janie's moods became extremely erratic. Her anxiety was unbearable.

Initially, Janie went back to her doctor to get refills. At some point, her primary care physician felt she was using too much medication and refused to refill her prescription as frequently as Janie requested. In her desperation to quell her anxiety, Janie began to seek out less orthodox means to obtain her sedatives. This behavior continued to escalate until she was in a state of full-blown dependence. Janie was able to hide her addiction from family and friends until she got into a car accident that could have had devastating consequences. Thankfully, Janie was not seriously hurt. The good that came out of this is that she finally got the help she needed.

Obsessive Compulsive Disorder

Obsessive Compulsive Disorder (OCD) is a disturbance in which an individual is plagued by intrusive, disturbing thoughts that the individual attempts to quell by engaging in meaningless, repetitive behaviors. The thoughts and the behaviors are accompanied by a significant degree of anxiety. Women who have suffered from (OCD) or obsessive-compulsive tendencies prior to the onset of perimenopause are at risk for increased symptoms once the hormonal changes of perimenopause begin.[152] Perimenopause brings a tri-fold increase in risk regarding OCD. The risk of developing OCD for the first time, the chance of OCD already present becoming more severe and the risk for the relapse of OCD that existed previously but was in remission, all increase with the onset of perimenopause.[153] The reason for this is that OCD is an anxiety-based disorder. When anxiety levels are increased, the vulnerability to this anxiety-fueled disorder is increased. We have already learned that anxiety levels increase in the perimenopausal woman as the levels of estrogen fluctuate and progesterone declines.

Camilla's Compulsion

Camilla's story is an example of how a number of factors came together during perimenopause resulting in a very distressing experience. Camilla has always struggled with OCD. She had a family history of OCD and initially began to show symptoms when she reached puberty. After the birth of each of her children, the OCD temporarily worsened until her hormones leveled out. As Camilla entered her forties, she began to suffer from anxiety with occasional bouts of depression. Still, she managed to run her life in a productive and fulfilling manner. She worked, raised her children and managed her household successfully.

In her middle forties, Camilla was in full-blown perimenopause. When she transitioned from Stage II, Emotional Disruption to Stage III, Turbulence, Camilla saw a spike in her OCD symptoms. She began to feel herself tangled in a torturous web as she became enslaved to her obsessive thoughts, washing her hands until her skin cracked and bled and fearing touching anything that was not "sanitary." Simultaneously, and not unrelated, Ca-

milla's moods deteriorated. Her anxiety was at an all time high, and she began to fall into deeply depressed moods. She started lashing out at her family until she had nearly destroyed her relationship with her children. Sadly, Camilla tried to manage her discomfort by turning to alcohol. Initially one drink was all she needed to feel better. In a short time, she needed to get drunk every day. It was not long before Camilla was completely immobilized by depression, OCD and alcoholism.

Panic Disorder

Panic Disorder, characterized by recurrent, persistent panic attacks is another disorder to which perimenopausal women are vulnerable. Similar to OCD, Panic Disorder is also an anxiety-based disorder. We have seen that anxiety, in general, worsens during the menopausal transition. The increased anxiety will promote the increased risk of developing Panic Disorder. The reduction in the amount of calming progesterone and the introduction of anxiety-producing hot flashes in the perimenopausal woman are believed to contribute to the increase of panic attacks in perimenopause.

The likelihood of suffering from Panic Disorder in perimenopause is greater in several circumstances. Women who have historically suffered from Panic Disorder will often experience a worsening of symptoms once they are in perimenopause. Those women with a family history of Panic Disorder will also be more likely to develop this disorder. The same vulnerability is there for women who suffered from panic attacks premenstrually or in the postpartum period.[154] Happily, once women enter their postmenopausal period, they return to the level of Panic Disorder they had before perimenopause.[155]

Interactive Effects

The symptoms of depressive disorders and anxiety disorders frequently increase during perimenopause and in the fifth and sixth decades of life. We have already learned about the many factors that exacerbate the symptoms of mood disorders and anxiety disorders, worsening the depression or anxiety that is already in place. These range from the hormonal effects of perimenopause to the social psychological challenges of women in this age range.

Unfortunately, during periods of dramatic hormonal change, the impact of symptoms and disorders can become complex and interactive, especially when there is concurrent psychosocial change. For example, as anxiety increases, so does the incidence of self-injurious behaviors (such as cutting and substance abuse), eating disorders, Panic Disorder and Obsessive Compulsive Disorder. Depression frequently emerges along with anxiety in perimenopause. Likewise, when depression sets in, anxiety is more likely to emerge or worsen. Other disturbances such as Bipolar Disorder, with much higher rates of depressive episodes and Schizophrenia also show a peak in the early perimenopausal years.[156] This creates a picture in which the issues affecting a perimenopausal woman can become very blurred. The best course of action for such a woman is to see help from a professional that is knowledgeable enough to disentangle the various aspects of her difficulty.

Chapter Twenty-two

Sexual Functioning–Who Has Run Off with My Libido?

*I*n a multiethnic sample of women questioned for the SWAN (Study of Women's Health across the Nation), 40 percent of women reported a low or absent desire for sex. In fact, the lack of sexual desire was the most frequent sexual complaint in women studied in several countries. Surprisingly, the majority of women studied *were* capable of arousal under the right circumstances,[157] but 50 to 60 percent of women between the ages of forty-two and fifty-two had difficulty with the intensity and frequency of orgasms.[158]

When we look at this shift in sexual desire and sexual functioning caused by perimenopause, we can see yet another challenge to a woman's sense of wellbeing during the menopausal transition. Many women find that their libido is far below what it was before perimenopause took hold. Researchers have found that in a study of over 300 women that 64 percent of peri- and postmenopausal women had diminished libido.[159] When one considers how many women are represented by this statistic, it is a large number of individual women struggling with their lack of sexual desire.

Libido Thieves

The mechanism by which arousal occurs in women is not well understood but is believed to be influenced by the interactive effects of neurotransmitters, sex hormones, psychological, and environmental factors. When female hormones run amok, the interaction between all of these factors combines with the unique difficulties of perimenopause, creating a complicated and confusing dynamic. How is a woman struggling with so many changes supposed to feel sexy, especially when she does not understand what is happening?

The foremost effect of perimenopause, the drop in estrogen and testosterone, are very significant for the plummeting libido.[160] The lower estrogen levels cause thinning and dryness in the vaginal tissues.[161] The lack of adequate lubrication in the lining of the vagina can cause irritation and pain, which is exacerbated during sexual activity.[162] Dyspareunia (painful intercourse) and a reduction in one's ability to be aroused are often the result.[163] These physiological changes in the vagina and surrounding tissues contribute to the plummeting sex drive and less sexual activity in perimenopause. Research has shown that one way to help compensate for the lubrication deficiency in the vagina caused by declining estrogen levels is to provide adequate sexual stimulation.[164] If women and their partners are aware of this, they can take measures to insure that sex can still be satisfying and enjoyable.

Another libido thief is the night sweat. The intrusiveness and frequency of some vasomotor symptoms, specifically night sweats that create mild to severe sleep disruption, are correlated with low libido and a diminished frequency of sex.[165] When a woman faces the nighttime with trepidation of having yet another sleepless night, her state of mind will unlikely be one conducive to relaxation and romance. Similarly, when she is exhausted from nights of disrupted sleep or night sweats, sex may begin to feel more like a chore for which she has not the energy or desire.

Other factors that can dampen libido and impact sexual functioning and performance are thyroid dysfunction, depression and anxiety, all of which are more prevalent during perimenopause than previously or afterwards. Decreased libido is much more prevalent in depressed women and in women who have insomnia. Because insomnia, vasomotor symptoms, and depression are so highly correlated, it can be difficult teasing apart the real culprit in declining sexual desire in women who are coping with a number of these issues.[166]

In addition to the physiological factors inhibiting libido, there are psychosocial and psychological factors. Once again, one must consider the interaction between the physiological and psychological factors. The relationship a woman has with her partner before she begins perimenopause, such as duration of the relationship, health of the relationship and the level of intimacy with a partner can influence how she manages her changing libido when in the perimenopausal transition. Perimenopause adds a new layer of discomfort that will be handled better if the relationship was strong and healthy previously. If the relationship is weak, flawed or there are unresolved difficulties from way back, they will likely rear up and become problematic when perimenopause gets underway. Women that have had a comfortable, emotionally intimate relationship with their partners will more likely be comfortable sharing with their partners the difficulties they are experiencing. When women can discuss their insecurities, the changes in their bodies, and the new and different ways their bodies respond sexually, they are better able to find solutions with their partners.

Women who lack emotional intimacy with their partners are more inclined to try and sort through and resolve the complications alone. Some women explain to themselves that the change in their sexual desire is due to a loss of interest in their partners. This puts increased distance between their partners and themselves. Such women and their partners are likely to wind up feeling isolated or even rejected. Difficulties escalate into dysfunctions when the concerns lay unaddressed and avoided. In the case of women, as opposed to men, the influence of such difficulties will more directly influence their sexual desire and responsivity. Men are left feeling confused and rejected while the women feel misunderstood.

Depression and Libido

The onset of depression, which is highly prevalent in perimenopause, has a very negative effect on libido. We have learned how debilitating depression can be. It will not only sap a woman's zest for life but will make small efforts seem monumental. A depressed woman who is continually tired, irritable and overwhelmed is unlikely to have a desire for sex. Conversely, a woman who is struggling with a flagging or absent sex drive may feel inadequate and fearful which may lead her towards depression.

Depression combined with the changes in a woman's body that in Western culture are typically viewed as negative, create a double challenge. The perimenopausal woman has probably gained a few pounds, more around the middle. Her breasts have lost some of their perkiness and she is sprouting chin hairs. When she looks in the mirror, her hair and skin have lost some luster, she sees more and more lines and some sagging skin. The thoughts and feelings associated with these perceptions will augment already depressed feelings and certainly will not make her feel sexy! Many women feel self conscious about these changes. What most women lose sight of is that the man in her life notices almost none of these physical changes. When he does notice, it is typically without the harsh negativity that women perceive. Most men report they do not care about these changes and see their women as desirous as ever. Let us not forget…men's bodies are changing, too!

Many perimenopausal women choose to take antidepressants to manage their labile moods. Unfortunately, this may create an additional challenge for sexual desire. Sexual disorders have been reported in as many as 58 percent of women taking antidepressants. Those taking SSRIs (a class of antidepressants) have even higher rates of sexual disorders,[167] some of whom will experience difficulty in achieving orgasm. This side effect is sometimes alleviated with the development of tolerance or dosage reduction. In some situations, other antidepressant classes that do not have the same effects on libido and sexuality as the SSRIs may be substituted.[168] If antidepressant medications are indicated for a perimenopausal woman, she and her doctor will need to discuss her individual needs and the side effects in order to find the right medication for her. There may be a bit of trial and error until the ideal match is made.

Time to Regroup

So where does all of this leave a woman? Her body has changed in uncountable ways. Physically, her skin and hair have changed. In all likelihood she has gained some weight and the weight has redistributed into a less "girlish" figure. Her digestion is slowed, leaving her a bit gassier and aside from being exhausted from her insomnia and night sweats, she only has to worry about her moods shifting on a dime. How is she supposed to feel sexy? Believe it or not, there are many ways in which women can find some relief in this area.

A woman in perimenopause can find calm and peace in ways that may be different than before. When she can achieve a measure of tranquility, she will be better able to access her sexual feelings. We explored earlier, in Chapter 14, how women come into the menopausal transition exhausted and depleted from a lifetime of giving to and doing for others. Her energy, both physically and psychologically, is at low ebb. Her self-confidence has taken a beating and it is tough to find ways to feel good about herself. This can present a wonderful and necessary opportunity to regroup-if she is willing to listen to her own needs.

Ronni's Lost Libido

Ronni squirmed, looking embarrassed and avoiding eye contact while her husband Bob complained that Ronni was never interested in sex anymore. Ronni held a stressful job and was a devoted mother to their autistic child. She was the "classic" peri-menopausal woman who felt unattractive due to her noticeable weight gain. She was exhausted from her many commitments and her hormones had absconded with her libido. She loved Bob but would have been content to be totally platonic. This did not sit well with Bob, who was beginning to wonder if Ronni's feelings towards him were changing. He even questioned if Ronni might be interested in another man.

While it is very frustrating and painful to struggle with diminished or absent sexual desire, it is important to remember that your sex drive will re-emerge. Working with your partner on what is and is not pleasurable is critical in getting through this time without relationship damage. Though you may not be inclined towards sexual activity, many perimenopausal women welcome and enjoy sensual activity. Sensual touching and stroking can be emotionally comforting. It will also cause the secretion of oxytocin, a hormone that calms and relaxes. Occasionally, such tender activities end up stimulating sexual desire. Even when this does not happen, it can bring a woman and her partner close in new and wonderful ways.

After Ronni and Bob got a thorough education on how perimenopause evolves and in particular, its effects on libido, they went home with some tips on how to reconnect with one another. Bob relaxed as he realized there was no need for concern regarding other love interests and that Ronni's lack of libido was a normal result of her changing hormones. Ronni felt less embarrassment and much less pressure to be sexual once the dynamics were understood by both of them. Several weeks later, Bob happily reported he had become quite adept at helping Ronni "produce oxytocin." He had become patient and understanding with Ronni especially since he felt he could help her through this transition. Ronni's stress eased as she realized how much Bob loved her, regardless of her extra weight, and how committed he was to their relationship.

This time offers women another wonderful opportunity- and that is to break the stronghold between external beauty and self-esteem. The

cultural drive to focus excessively on weight and appearance as a determination of "sexiness" needs to change. It is as impossible to prevent the
changes in our perimenopausal bodies, as it was to prevent the changes
of puberty. Our bodies are just as beautiful (and as attractive to men)
as they ever were. We are just beautiful in a different, more mature
way. We can use our new bodies, our hearts and our minds together to
evaluate our sense of self and self-confidence. We can reorganize and
reprioritize our lives such that we can feel good about ourselves. We can
focus on ourselves and connect with what gives us pleasure and fulfillment. All of these changes will allow for our sensuality and sexuality to
take on new life.

Chapter Twenty-three

The Emotional Blender

Who is the forty- to fifty-something year old, perimenopausal woman? Is she an undiagnosed case of Attention Deficit Disorder? After all, she cannot seem to remember a thing anymore, her concentration lasts approximately a half minute and she gets lost trying to sort through the simplest of concepts. Is she really a lazy person, who just never got around to being lazy before? Suddenly all she really wants to do is lie on the couch eating carbohydrates and watching television. She really does not care if the laundry is done or her work is finished. Is she the beleaguered wife who never realized she just could not stand her husband? She has no interest in sex and finds him annoying in just about *everything* he says and does. Is she the bad mother who just cannot muster up her previous levels of concern for and involvement in her children's lives? Is she the closet sociopath? Everyone and everything seems so ridiculous. She does not have patience for all of the nonsense.

She gains weight easily and her waist is thickening. She is aging. She is tired. She is anxious. She is depressed. She has no energy. Nothing has the same meaning as it did *before*. She no longer knows who she is. She may turn to alcohol. She may abuse prescription medication. She may shut out everything in the throes of depression or she may rage at the world in fits of anxiety.

The term "Emotional Blender" refers to the subjective experience of swirling, confusing feelings, lack of self-understanding and the sense of being utterly unfamiliar with oneself that is so characteristic of these women. The overall picture of herself is chaotic. What is different? Perhaps it is everything. Perhaps it is nothing. We know for sure that everything *feels* different. That is one of the most disconcerting aspects of this transition. By the time women enter their forties, they feel they know who they are. Along comes perimenopause and everything they thought they knew about themselves becomes upended.

Women who believed they had figured out their own optimal way of living life suddenly find it is no longer satisfying. This can be any woman. It can be the woman who always knew she wanted to stay home and raise her children. Suddenly, this is not fulfilling and she begins to wonder if she should have developed a career. It can be the woman like Diana, who built a lucrative career as a physician. Diana hit her mid-forties, gave up her practice and chose to be home so she could carpool and help with homework like all of the other moms. By the time Diana had reached fifty, and the end of perimenopause, she was back to practicing medicine. It can be the woman like Elisha who searches for an activity, any activity she might enjoy but finds every one unappealing.

While the experience of every woman is unique, there is one thread that ties together most women; that for each of them life feels more confusing and conflicted than ever before. One fifty year old woman, Kim, who was just finishing Stage III, Turbulence and happened to be a feminist said to me, "I hate to say this, but I am not sure women in this stage of life should hold important offices." What Kim was trying to convey was that in her experience, women often strayed so far from who they were previously that there was a question as to whether they could trust their own judgment. It is for this reason that I will usually recommend that while in the most difficult stages of perimenopause, Stages II and III, Emotional Disruption and Turbulence, women delay making drastic or irrevocable life decisions. I have seen many women compelled to make a very disruptive choice while affected by the emotional chaos of this time who later on felt very different about the same issue, as was the case with Joanne.

Resentment Run Amok

Joanne was a stay at home mom. She had four children, a wonderful husband, a nice home and good friends. She was active in the community and in her children's schools. Her husband was a successful attorney who made a good living, enabling Joanne to be home without the concern for bringing in a second income. Joanne's life was storybook perfect until she hit perimenopause.

The first sign that things were changing was when Joanne's oldest child began getting ready to find a college. Joanne and her daughter became embroiled in conflict that spilled over into all of the family dynamics. Joanne began to feel that her insides were constantly churning. Soon, Joanne and her husband began arguing. Joanne felt that her husband, Paul was not supportive enough. Before long, the other three children were feeling and engaging in the tension that was disrupting the entire household. Joanne began to resent Paul for things that had never before been an issue. She was scornful if he neglected to pick up something at the supermarket. She was angry if he put the meat in the freezer instead of the refrigerator. She felt betrayed if he tried to intervene in problems with the children and felt alone if he did not. It got to the point that Joanne could not stand the sight of Paul. Paul felt that no matter what efforts he made, there was no pleasing Joanne.

Joanne began to lose interest in sex while simultaneously rapidly gaining weight. Her cravings for sweets and carbohydrates were out of control, as was her willpower to avoid eating them.

Dieting was useless. Joanne was simply unable to lose weight. Most days left Joanne feeling miserable: tired, angry, unattractive, resentful or depressed. Joanne projected the cause of these feelings onto Paul; truly believing it was he that was the source of her misery. Unfortunately for Joanne and her husband, neither was very aware or insightful about the internal changes Joanne was experiencing. Joanne was considering ending her marriage when she sought help. By the time Joanne completed her menopausal transition, she and Paul had resumed their harmonious relationship.

Women will respond differently to the physical and emotional changes that are coursing through them. Different personality traits will produce varying responses. Women who tend to turn inward when facing difficulty may be more inclined towards depression or anxiety. Women who are more outwardly expressive may exhibit anger or rage. Whether directed inwardly or outwardly, the frenetic chaos of the hormonally induced emotional typhoon is very difficult to manage, especially when women and their loved ones do not understand what is happening.

The place where a woman is in her life cycle is another significant factor that affects her ability to cope in this transition. Women who started their families at older ages may face perimenopause while having young children to take care of. The challenge for these women is that with young children one does not have as much latitude for error. Young children are unable to understand mom's unpredictability the way an older child may. An irrational rage or breakdown is much easier to explain to an older child. A young child simply does not have the maturity or coping mechanisms to understand. This places additional pressure on mom to try to balance what is nearly impossible to balance. Add to this the difficulty in getting some time alone to decompress when your children are small and the strain can become unbearable.

If your children are pubescent when you are also hormonal, you can expect some real fireworks. You will both be at the mercy of fluctuating and unpredictable hormonal states. You will seek the comfort and understanding of the other, while each will be depleted of the ability to give it. If your children are older, you have the changing dynamics of children leaving the nest to contend with.

Distinct miseries arise in women who have not had children but had always hoped to. The end of fertility for these women is exceptionally painful. These women have to psychologically negotiate the ending of a lifelong desire. This creates a unique and significant risk of depression.

Any substantial adversity, whether it is the ending of a relationship, death or illness in a loved one or oneself or even a catastrophic job or financial upheaval, will be far less manageable and infinitely more painful during the perimenopausal juncture.

Each of these situations presents its unique hardships. Each contributes to the already unpleasant and unmanageable torrent of emotions in perimenopause. Hopefully, in knowing that the emotional chaos of perimenopause is a normal part of an inescapable life transition, women will find the strength to muddle through while keeping their families healthy and intact. Having the support of informed family members is of priceless value. Part IV is dedicated to this understanding.

Chapter Twenty-four

Finding a Way Out

$\mathscr{N}$ ow that we have an understanding of the many difficulties and the significant distress perimenopausal women
endure, we need to find a way in which we can alleviate these miseries.
Unfortunately, many women get lost in the overwhelming nature of what
they are struggling with and how to choose the best treatment options.
There is a lot of confusing information that offers conflicting advice. The
following section will untangle much of the confusion by exploring the
available treatment options including hormonal treatment, supplements,
psychotropic medication, energy and mind-body therapies. Final decisions on all medical treatments should always be made in conjunction
with a qualified health care provider who has reasonable knowledge and
understanding of your particular needs.

Treatment Options

Hormonal Treatment

One of the dilemmas women with severe perimenopausal symptoms face is whether or not to use what is commonly referred to as HRT

(hormone replacement therapy). Since "HRT" is only a partial "replacement," more accurately a substitution of hormones, it is more accurate to refer to it as "hormone therapy" or "HT". HT is the administration of synthetic or animal estrogens and progesterone and was the typical treatment modality for perimenopause and menopause related symptoms until the early 2000s. The reason HT was so popular in perimenopausal women is that estrogen replacement improves cognitive functioning, especially verbal skills and memory, reduces the risk of Alzheimer's Disease and reduces depression.[169] It also diminishes vasomotor symptoms and improves irregular bleeding patterns.[170] Estrogen combined with progesterone therapy also reduces depression in perimenopausal women.[171] It was a miracle solution for this difficult transition.

In 2002, the WHI (Women's Health Initiative), a comprehensive government sponsored fifteen year study on HT, was cancelled four years early because of the adverse effects women were suffering from taking these hormones. The study results showed an increased risk of heart attack, stroke, breast cancer and pulmonary embolism in the women who took the synthetic estrogen and progestin. Since that time doctors are reluctant to prescribe this type of treatment and wisely, women are very frightened to take it, leaving women to find alternate ways to ameliorate unpleasant perimenopausal symptoms.[172]

Thankfully, researchers were already exploring an alternate method of managing and replacing female hormones in perimenopause by using bioidentical hormones. Bioidentical hormones are identical in molecular structure to the hormones naturally made in a woman's body. Bioidentical estrogens are extracted from substances in yams and soy and are called phytoestrogens. Bioidentical progesterone is simply micronized progesterone, often made from wild yams. Bioidentical hormones behave in the body in identical ways to what the body manufactures and are indistinguishable on blood tests from the hormones the body creates.

It is believed that bioidentical hormones are much safer than synthetic or animal hormones for overall health. It is known that they can effectively treat many of the disruptive symptoms of perimenopause.

Bioidentical estrogen reduces depression,[173] helps minimize mood swings and can even reduce wrinkles when applied topically.[174] Bioidentical estradiol (one of the three estrogens) significantly reduces the severity and frequency of hot flashes.[175] Because phytoestrogens are present in food sources, it is easy to add them to your diet. By taking supplements or eating a diet rich in phytoestrogens a woman can increase the amount of bioidentical estrogens in her body. If she prefers, she can use a pill, transdermal cream, patch, nasal spray or vaginal cream instead or in addition to food sources.

Bioidentical progesterone is also extremely helpful in managing peri-menopausal symptoms, again, without the risk of synthetic hormones. It promotes calm, reduces depression, increases bone density, supports thyroid hormone and balances estrogen.[176] Additionally, it is beneficial in managing heavy menstrual flow and breast tenderness.[177] Perhaps the most appreciated effect of bioidentical progesterone is that it improves sleep (especially when taken orally or intravaginally). It also alleviates anxiety and mood swings, perks up libido and will reduce hot flashes and night sweats.[178]

Typically, bioidentical progesterone is administered by using a trans-dermal cream. It is simple, easy to use and most of all, effective. Many women make the transition from miserable to bearable simply by using bioidentical progesterone cream. Its effectiveness in easing many peri-menopausal symptoms cannot be underestimated. One woman, Margo, was losing the battle with her perimenopausal symptoms primarily be-cause of her profound exhaustion. A week after she began using a com-pounded preparation of bioidentical progesterone, she was sleeping bet-ter and hence able to tolerate her moodiness and irritability.

Two other bioidentical hormones are worth mentioning. Since tes-tosterone and DHEA levels also decrease in women in their forties and fif-ties, supplementing them can produce a number of benefits. Bioidentical testosterone and DHEA (a precursor to testosterone) help revive libido, prevent against bone loss, and increase energy and alertness. DHEA and bioidentical progesterone both have strong anti-carcinogenic properties, so they are beneficial for perimenopausal women with cancer risks.[179] With the proper supplementation of the hormones that are reduced during perimenopause, women can mitigate many of the disruptive symptoms that wreak havoc in their lives without taking unnecessary risks of getting other medical problems by using synthetic hormones.

Psychotropic Medications

A different approach to managing the unpleasant symptoms of perimenopause is using psychotropic medications: anxiolytics, antidepressants or hypnotics (sleep aids). The reason these nonhormonal medications may be the treatment of choice is that they do not have the risks that HT has. They alleviate many perimenopausal and life stage induced troubles while producing minimal side effects. New research shows impressive benefits of these medications. For example, escitalopram (brand name Lexapro), traditionally used as an antidepressant medication with anxiolytic properties, has been found to reduce by over 50 percent, hot flash frequency and severity in perimenopausal women, even in women with no depression or anxiety.[180] This same medication effectively decreases depression and anxiety and improves libido in women who are struggling with those symptoms.[181] For the symptomatic, perimenopausal woman, this one medication can relieve a wide range of difficulties.

Other psychotropic medications, paroxetine (brand name Paxil—used for anxiety, panic and depression), venlafaxine (brand name Effexor—used for depression and GAD), clonidine (used for hypertension and insomnia)[182] and gabapentin (brand name Neurontin—used for seizures and pain reduction) have all shown promise for relief of vasomotor symptoms[183, 184] in addition to their primary purposes. Eszopiclone (brand name Lunesta) is a sedative, typically prescribed for insomnia. Recently, this too, has revealed an impressive effect on some of the symptoms of perimenopause. Eszopiclone not only relieves insomnia, it can also reduce depression, anxiety, night sweats and improves overall quality of life.[185]

Many women are reluctant to take sleep medications for fear of dependency. While caution is always advised before starting any type of medication, it is critical to consider the benefits of adequate sleep before refusing such an intervention. I refer you back to Chapter 9 where the potentially devastating ripple effect of compounded sleep deprivation was established. Sleep is the ultimate healer and restorer of good health. Using pharmaceuticals to restore sleep at this difficult juncture in life is preferable to accumulating a huge sleep deficit with its accompanying misery. The combined benefit of reducing mood disorders, vasomotor symptoms and even improving sleep disruption is encouraging more women to try these nonhormonal medications as the first and best therapy for the many challenges they face at this time of life. In most cases treatment with medication is required only until the worst of perimenopause has passed.

Camilla's Solution

In Chapter 21 we met Camilla. She had fallen into a pattern of abusing alcohol after her OCD spiked in perimenopause. Camilla's story ended well. After discontinuing her dependence on alcohol, Camilla was given psychotropic medication to manage her anxiety, depression and OCD. As she felt better, she returned to a structured exercise program that she had given up two years prior. Her psychological symptoms virtually disappeared and Camilla began feeling better and acting better. The most destructive of her perimenopausal symptoms were alleviated with these medications making it unnecessary for her to consider taking HT. It took some time but Camilla was able to repair the damage done in her relationships and rebuild trust with her family. The remainder of perimenopause was very manageable for Camilla.

Supplements

Supplements can be used instead of or in conjunction with other treatments. Many of the supplements available for the reduction of perimenopausal symptoms include some type of phytoestrogen. Phytoestrogens are compounds that behave like estrogen in the body and are found in plants, fruits and vegetables. While they are much weaker than human estrogen, they bind to estrogen receptors producing estrogen-like effects. They also have anti-estrogenic effects[186] which makes them beneficial for managing perimenopausal difficulties. What is the mechanism by which this works? When estrogen levels are too high, phytoestrogen binds to the estrogen receptors, blocking the estrogen from binding. This reduces the effects of excess estrogen that we learned about in the first chapter. When there is not enough estrogen, phytoestrogen binds to the estrogen receptors, behaving like estrogen, mitigating the effects of low estrogen.

The types of phytoestrogens include:

- Isoflavones, the most potent of the phytoestrogens (found in soy and legumes),
- Lignans (found in flaxseed, beans, fruits, vegetables and whole grains), and
- Coumestans (found in sprouting plants and red clover).

The isoflavones, genistein and daidzein are the most commonly used phytoestrogen supplements. Women have a host of choices for getting more of these helpful nutrients into their systems. The availability of soy products has mushroomed in recent years. Anything "soy"—soy milk, powder, protein, drink or bean will all add phytoestrogens. If you cannot tolerate soy food products, the other food choices listed above will suffice or you may prefer to supplement with phytoestrogen capsules or pills.

Research has demonstrated that once phytoestrogens are in the body, they mimic many of the benefits of estrogen for the perimenopausal woman. Such benefits include improving cognitive functioning and reducing the frequency and severity of vasomotor events.[187, 188] They also alleviate irritability, depression, loss of libido, insomnia and headaches.[189] Phytoestrogens have benefits that exceed those that are just for perimenopausal symptoms. For example, they have anti-carcinogenic properties, reducing risks for developing breast cancer[190] and colon cancer. They also reduce the risks of heart disease[191] and osteoporosis. We are only just beginning to understand the breadth of the advantages this natural food-based substance can offer for our health and wellbeing.

Similar to the benefits of phytoestrogens, black cohosh is a supplement that has been proven to relieve many perimenopausal symptoms. Women in research studies who were given black cohosh experienced a reduction or resolution of many symptoms including hot flashes, night sweats, insomnia, headaches, vaginal dryness, fatigue, mood swings, and irritability.[192, 193]

There are several supplements not specifically marketed to perimenopausal women that can be of significant benefit during this transition. Phospholipid liposomes (lecithin is the most popular phospholipid) has shown great promise in reducing anxiety, dizziness, restlessness, weakness and depression in perimenopausal women.[194] Adding evening primrose oil and vitamin E supplements to your diet will relieve hot flashes. Melatonin may offer you some relief if you are one of the many perimenopausal women who awakens exhausted, depressed and ready for your daily cry in the shower. Melatonin improves sleep, can have a positive effect on mood and increases levels of thyroid hormone in perimenopausal women[195] (see Chapter 26 for the incidence and effects of low thyroid levels in perimenopause).

Energy Therapy

Acupuncture has gained a lot of interest as an effective treatment option for perimenopausal and postmenopausal women. It has shown efficacy in reducing the intensity and frequency of vasomotor symptoms by half. It improves sleep (more so by the reduction of night sweats), and eases somatic symptoms such as joint and limb pain, headaches, abdominal pain, back pain and discomfort in the breasts.[196] Studies have shown that after only four weeks of acupuncture, women can see a decrease in feelings of depression, irritability, anxiety, aggressiveness, mental exhaustion, forgetfulness, bladder problems and vaginal discomfort.[197]

Acupuncture is reasonably priced, easy to administer, has no side effects, and best of all, it works! If you have problems with needles, acupressure can be just as effective.[198]

Mind-Body Therapies

Relaxation breathing, meditation, progressive muscle relaxation, aerobic exercise and yoga have all shown beneficial effects in perimenopausal women.[199] Research on yoga has shown positive changes in heart rate, breathing, blood pressure and psychological symptoms.[200] Perimenopausal women who practice yoga have shown a reduction in a wide variety of perimenopausal complaints. Vasomotor symptoms, psychological symptoms including perceived stress, anxiety, depression, fatigue, and neuroticism all improved when put on yoga regimens in various studies.[201] There are similar positive changes in women practicing meditation.[202]

Exercise is another healthy way to reduce perimenopausal symptoms. As little as twenty minutes of exercise three times a week can reduce hot flashes.[203] Even an easy exercise routine that does not cause sweating has been shown to improve vasomotor symptoms, improve psychological wellbeing and reduce stressful feelings.[204] If that is not enough motivation, it will also help with that mid-life weight gain while giving you a healthy dose of those wonderful endorphins!

Keep in mind that any "therapy" that you would ordinarily find soothing will help in perimenopause. Whether your preference is for massage, relaxation breathing, progressive muscle relaxation, music, meditation or painting walls, if it helps you to calm down, it will be beneficial during this transition. Many women find it useful to listen to relaxation tapes, use aroma therapy, or just spend a day every so often at a spa. A practice as simple as paced respiration, a method of slowing one's breathing, can even relieve the unpleasant symptoms of hot flashes.[205]

Finding activities that help you to decompress or just take a break from "life" will make it easier to relax and to sleep, helping you to be more resistant to the many symptoms that assault women during perimenopause. You can find your own optimal results by trying a combination of various therapies. This is a time for self-nurturance and self care. It is too easy to get lost in a hopeless place when women neglect what they need. This is the one time of life that women cannot afford to put themselves last. Keep in mind that when you are better, others you care about will benefit; when you are lost, they will suffer, too.

Last but not least, psychotherapy, whether it is in the style of individual, group or support group therapy, is an extremely effective tool in wading through the ups and downs of this transition. Individual psychotherapy helps women cope with their personal challenges in a one-to-one encounter. When using a psychologist who is knowledgeable about perimenopause and issues pertaining to women in this age range, a woman can learn how current challenges are woven into the whole fabric of who she is—past and present. This is helpful in alleviating depression and anxiety, will improve her general sense of wellbeing and facilitate coping with current and new challenges.

Group therapy or support groups focus more on the mutual support of participants than on the relationship between the patient and therapist. Typically this forum will concentrate on a singular topic that unites the participants who will share personal experiences and information. Research has proven that women who are more educated and knowledgeable about what is happening to them fare much better.

Educating Lori

The case of Lori shows how important knowledge and understanding can be. Lori was forty-five when she initially came for therapy. She was severely depressed, highly anxious, had trouble sleeping and felt like she was coming apart. She was taking sick leave from work due to her emotional state. When questioned, Lori did not have any specific event or crisis pointing to her current emotional chaos. Her marriage was healthy, her children happy, she had typical ups and downs with her mother and sibling and she hated her job; nothing out of the ordinary.

I began to explore with Lori whether this might be hormonally induced, suspecting the perimenopause culprit. Lori looked at me as if I was crazy. Lori had never paid much attention to "menopause issues"; she was way too young for that! This was my cue to give Lori some information. As I began to explain perimenopause to Lori, the mood swings, the insomnia, relationship shifts, identity struggles, fatigue, libido changes and all else, I saw the shock and simultaneous relief in Lori's face. As I described each of these symptoms, Lori was nodding and recognizing herself in my words.

The truth was, Lori was right in the middle of Turbulence. Relief swept through her as soon as she had a context in which to understand herself. Lori and I continued to work together as she passed through her remaining stages of perimenopause. She had her difficult moments but through this new understanding she was able to make changes in her life that would facilitate the process. What always stuck with me was the question Lori asked me at the end of her first session… "Why doesn't everyone know about all of this perimenopause stuff?"

Where to Begin?

With so many treatment options, where does one begin? Many women in this stage of life find themselves with multiple challenges, as we have learned. The question of what sort of medical professional to start with can be as confusing as determining what treatment options to pursue. Psychiatrists will be qualified to prescribe medication for depression and anxiety, but it is unlikely they will be able to address thyroid related mood issues or hormonal issues resulting from perimenopause. The endocrinologist can certainly treat the thyroid, but little else. A woman's gynecologist may not be competent in interpreting all of the psychological symptoms nor in educating and treating the woman for the complex psychological/perimenopausal issues. Research has shown that male physicians are much less likely to identify depression in their female patients than are female physicians, so depression in patients with male doctors may be completely missed. Most psychologists are certainly trained to help a woman cope with her anxiety, depression, mood fluctuations and life events, but few are extremely knowledgeable about the physiological components of her troubles and how they interact with psychological events. The difficulty finding the practitioners that can give women the answers they need can deepen their distress and overwhelm them.

The best option for women with multiple issues is to develop a multi-faceted approach to feeling better. A "team approach" will offer the most successful outcome. More than one specialist may be required to bring a woman to her optimal level of functioning. It is important when choosing doctors and health practitioners that women find those who are willing to communicate with one another and work together on her behalf. It is also beneficial to seek health professionals who are open-minded in trying alternative approaches as a means to achieve mind/body health. Asking the practitioner before getting started if they are willing to meet your requirements, will save you from much frustration and disappointment later.

Fortunately, there is a wealth of research emerging on the many ways in which to feel better at this time of life, enlightening and educating more health practitioners. Perhaps most important is to become informed and to talk with others. One woman found that while working out at the gym on seniors' day she met many older women who were happy to share their experiences and wisdom with her. This unique approach gave her great comfort since she was not able to have such discussions with her own mother. Friends, family, coworkers, the saleswoman at your favorite store are all potential sources of information and referrals. The best results often come from a personal story and learning how someone else found solutions.

Self Care

This is your time to ask friends and family for their help, support, understanding and patience. Rather than nurture everyone else first, consider yourself first, and invite others to nurture you. The transition through perimenopause is a unique opportunity for women to grow and develop. Women accomplish this most easily by embracing the many physical and emotional changes instead of fighting them. Exploring new methods of engaging with the same old situations allows evolution of the self. This will bring forth a new perspective and a whole new sense of power. Experiment with releasing some of the tired old responsibilities and allow new interests to evolve and take root. With the right balance of emotional, medical and physiological interventions with self-care, the passage through perimenopause will bring women into a wonderful new era of their lives.

Chapter Twenty-five

After the Storm

What happens after a woman transitions through perimenopause? Her hormones have quieted down. The storm of unpredictably changing emotions has passed. Who is she now? This is a time of redefinition. From the simplest to the most complex issues, she is changed. For some 40 years, her existence was divided into monthly cycles. Menstruation is a marker of time, of sexuality, of fertility and of mood. Even in someone whose cycles were not too intrusive, a woman was aware of when she should not book that tropical vacation, so as not to coincide with her period. She knew if this was her fertile week or the week she might be premenstrual and feeling below par. Now, this is no longer the case. Even on this very simplistic level, her life is fundamentally changed.

One of the most obvious changes is that the postmenopausal woman has to redefine herself as no longer fertile. For some women, this is an enormous relief. They feel freer to enjoy sex without the worries of pregnancy, especially after the last years when menstruation was so irregular. For other women, there is sadness, a mourning of sorts for the end of their reproductive capabilities. Some women, as they approach this deadline, suddenly begin to reconsider whether they might want another child "before it is too late." This is usually a momentary wistful thought. An image of a soft, sweet newborn can be tantalizing until one thinks of exhaustive days and nights caring for one. The yearnings, the relief and the freedoms all contribute to the reconciliation of the end of the fertile period of life.

Fortunately, most women feel a tremendously positive sense of promise as they begin this new era. This shift begins before menopause as women enter Stage IV of perimenopause, Quietitude. Even those women who approached the end of their child rearing years with enormous trepidation can experience a newfound freedom and new potential unfolding in front of them. With the roller coaster of emotions that marked their perimenopausal years behind them, their female hormones diminish to a steady purr and the depression and anxiety ease.

In stark contrast to the chaos of the previous decade there is now a new sense of stability. Women can begin to explore new avenues and prospects that they lacked time and energy for in prior years. This is the time when women have the emotional resources to reinvent themselves. If they still have children at home, they will find themselves calmer with more patience and tolerance than in prior years. If the children have left the nest, women have a whole new world to explore and embrace, similar to how it was before they started their families.

Catherine's Evolution

Catherine's story is a wonderful example of how one woman evolved throughout her perimenopausal transition. Catherine began perimenopause in her mid-forties, shortly after her divorce. She had two teenagers at home, a sixteen year old daughter with whom she was very close, and a son who was a few years younger. Since Catherine had only worked part time jobs during the child rearing years, she began to anticipate with trepidation what the years ahead would bring once her children would be in college.

As the years passed and Catherine entered the second and third stages of perimenopause, Emotional Disruption and Turbulence, she suffered from depression regarding her status as a divorcee, anxiety about how she would be able to cope and feel fulfilled after her children would both be gone and rage at her ex-husband who always seemed to "have it so easy." Catherine was on an emotional roller coaster almost daily. Some days were so bad, especially the year her daughter left for college, that Catherine barely got off the couch. She decided to frenetically search for a mate who would solve all of her problems. If she could have a relationship established before her son left for college, all would be fine.

It did not take long before Catherine realized this was not the solution. As her son left for college, she was sliding into Quietude, the final stage of perimenopause. She was no longer at the mercy of her erratic emotional state. Catherine began to experience a vaguely familiar connection to the logical, goal- directed woman she was before perimenopause. Catherine took a step back from dating and decided to focus on her interests and find her passions. She realized this was her time now, to do what she wanted, when and how she wanted to do whatever it might be. Without the emotional and sleep-deprived veil of perimenopause that left Catherine unable to concentrate or plan her future, Catherine was able to make life decisions. She returned to school, launched herself into a new career and eventually decided to sell her large and burdensome home. She felt content and confident in a way that had eluded her in her younger years. This was her recipe for fulfillment.

As we can see in Catherine's story, a woman can begin a new life. It is one in which the old ties that bound her are let go, from the attachment to a monthly cycle to the ever-pressing demands of motherhood, career, community and serving everyone else's needs before her own. She can then assimilate new opportunities in which structure and obligation are less critical, a life in which she has more time and a fresh new sense of self-concern and self-care. This process allows her to become acquainted with a new sense of purpose and power. Although she may still experience bothersome vasomotor events, she will feel emotionally quiet. Gone is the swirling, churning emotional storm. In its place is stillness and emotional self-understanding. Depression and anxiety decline,[206] while cognition improves.[207] There is a recognition dawning on the postmenopausal woman that now life can be for her. She can revamp her love life, whether it is reconnecting with her husband or striking out with someone new. She can indulge in friendships with other women and explore the interests for which she never before had the time or patience. She can take that art class or learn tennis or take some courses at the local college. She can begin a new career or even write a book. This is her time, for the first time, in a long time.

Part III
PERIMENOPAUSE AND INCREASED RISK OF THYROID DISEASE: DISCOVERING THE HIDDEN TROUBLE MAKER

The prevalence of thyroid disease skyrockets in perimenopausal women. The thyroid is a butterfly shaped endocrine gland that sits at the base of the neck. It is the master gland for the body's metabolism through the hormones it produces. It regulates temperature, stress, sleep patterns, energy, brain, heart and other organ functions.

Hypothyroidism, more prevalent than hyperthyroidism, affects as much as 10 percent of women in the U.S. general population. With the onset of perimenopause, existing sufferers many have a more difficult time managing their disorder while women who previously were not diagnosed with thyroid disease may begin to notice symptoms. In both cases we may see a significant rise in depression and anxiety as a result of an inadequately functioning metabolism and endocrine system.

I dedicate these chapters to discussing the complex relationship between thyroid disease and perimenopause. Not insignificantly, many of the symptoms of thyroid disease are the same as or similar to those of perimenopause. Because symptoms overlap, it is imperative for a woman to recognize other possible causes for the changes occurring in her body if she is to address the issues properly.

Chapter Twenty-six

Hypothyroidism–Understanding the Metabolic, Physical, Cognitive and Emotional Changes

An important medical issue that is seen frequently in perimenopausal women is the development of thyroid disease, more typically hypothyroidism (underactive thyroid function). In the general population, hypothyroidism is one of the most common medical problems affecting women in this country with as many as 10 percent[208] in the general population and 26 percent of women over sixty years of age. Thyroid disease, especially hypothyroidism increases with age.[209] This disorder can range from mild to severe, with severe cases being quite debilitating. Women have a higher risk for developing hypothyroidism especially when there is a family history of thyroid disease, or if they suffer from an autoimmune disease.[210]

Because hypothyroidism is such a common phenomenon in women, especially as they enter their forties and fifties, and because the symptoms of hypothyroidism are so similar to those of perimenopause, it can be easily overlooked in the face of the hormonal changes of perimenopause. Hence, women need to become knowledgeable about the symptoms of thyroid disease in order to get the medical care that most accurately addresses their problems. Too often hypothyroidism is misdiagnosed because the symptoms are attributed to other problems. The symptoms of thyroid disease fall into four major categories: metabolic, physical, cognitive, and emotional.

Metabolic Symptoms

The most obvious symptoms felt by women who are hypothyroid are fatigue and lethargy. Heather noticed that in recent months she was feeling exhausted and had a sense of general malaise that was not relieved by one or many nights of adequate sleep. Unbeknownst to Heather, she had become hypothyroid. Her exhaustion was primarily explained by her thyroid's flagging ability to regulate her metabolism and energy. When the thyroid is underactive, energy declines. In addition to the lack of energy, the hypothyroid women, although tired, will not achieve the most restful and deep sleep (Stage 4 sleep). So, even though Heather was getting an average of 8 or more hours of sleep, her body was not rejuvenating itself during the nighttime hours. Together, these symptoms create the lethargy so characteristic of hypothyroidism.

Many people are aware that those with malfunctioning thyroids will be prone to weight gain. Hypothyroid women have trouble losing weight or will gain weight, regardless of diet. As Heather put on weight, she reduced her food intake, ate healthier with low calorie foods and still experienced difficulty in controlling her weight.[211] Women with struggling thyroids not only have slowed food metabolism, they also suffer from slowed bowel function, resulting in constipation.

The hypothyroid woman also suffers from a higher risk for cardiovascular disease as her pulse rate slows to between forty-five and sixty beats per minute, while her blood pressure is likely to increase. Due to her slowed metabolism, she will often feel cold or chilled, requiring heavy sweaters, even when those around her are warm or even hot. Hypothyroidism that is profound or prolonged can negatively impact cholesterol levels, as well. Together, these symptoms, when severe and untreated can put an individual at risk for heart attack and stroke. As soon as the hypothyroidism is treated and the individual is returned to a euthyroid state (a state of normal thyroid functioning), an otherwise healthy individual will return to their prior state of heart health and/or risk.[212]

Women with hypothyroidism will also suffer effects in menstruation. They will have changes in their menstrual cycles with irregular periods and an atypically heavy flow.[213, 214] They may develop fertility problems if the hypothyroidism causes anovulatory cycles. As we have already noted, when women age and enter perimenopause the risk of becoming hypothyroid increases. The inverse is also true. An unhealthy thyroid has been shown in reproductive endocrine studies to be a contributor to fluctuations in hormone levels that are implicit in the transition into menopause.[215]

It is apparent that many of the metabolic symptoms present in hypothyroidism are also present in perimenopause. Fatigue and lethargy are characteristic traits of both conditions. Again, in both hypothyroidism and perimenopause, women struggle with weight gain and difficulty in losing weight in a way that has previously not been typical for them. Digestion is slowed along with bowel function and can produce abdominal bloating and discomfort. The risk of cardiovascular disease increases in both of these populations, and finally, there is a definitive change in the menstrual cycle and menstrual flow in both conditions.

In hypothyroid women and in perimenopausal woman there may be anovulatory menstrual cycles, which create many of the problems described in Chapter 6. One very discerning difference between these two conditions is body temperature. In perimenopause, women are prone to feeling overheated but with hypothyroidism, women will feel cold. This is an important factor in differentiating between thyroid and perimenopause symptoms.

Physical Symptoms

The physical changes in hypothyroid women can be very distressing. One of the most obvious and more upsetting symptoms is thinning hair. Heather was appalled one morning when she saw clumps of hair falling out in her hairbrush. She also had recently noticed hair falling out in the shower and on her pillow. This was caused by her hypothyroidism. When hair loss is substantial, the hypothyroid women may find areas on her scalp that are thin to the point of balding. In Heather's case, as is common, her nails became brittle, easily breaking and peeling while new growth was very slow. Heather also began suffering from dry, flaky skin that was not eased by moisturizing and was dismayed to see puffiness and swelling in her face and around her eyes. Not only did she *feel* different, she *looked* different.

Other physical changes include muscle spasms and muscular weakness. Frequently the hypothyroid woman feels achy and her muscles are sore and painful. Hands and feet may tingle and be cold. Physical activity becomes much more difficult. She will be short of breath, finding herself huffing and puffing when applying a minimal physical effort. The same level of physical exertion that was once easily accomplished is an overwhelming endeavor in the hypothyroid woman. Recovery from physical exertion takes longer and is more difficult, often resulting in muscle or joint soreness or even chest pain. Her pulse may be slowed and her body temperature may be lower than 98.6 degrees.

Here again, in the domain of physical symptoms, we see the similarity between some of the symptoms of hypothyroidism and perimenopause. The dry, lackluster skin is common to both conditions. Hair loss and brittle nails are also common to both. The aches and pains in joints and muscles combine with the challenges of physical exertion to augment lethargy and create a state of feeling poorly.

The differences, again, are as important to notice as are the similarities. Body temperature is low in hypothyroidism; in perimenopause it is normal. Additionally, while both conditions are characterized by lethargy, in hypothyroidism, especially when it is severe, the exhaustion will be much more debilitating than in perimenopause (unless the perimeno-pausal woman is also suffering from depression).

Cognitive Symptoms

As Heather's hypothyroidism took hold, she began noticing changes in her concentration and memory. The cognitive changes that are caused by hypothyroidism can be very frightening. Concentrating can become a Herculean task when there is a lack of thyroid hormone.[216, 217] Memory also shows a distinct lack of performance compared to how it was before there was a thyroid problem.[218] When forgetfulness accompanies a lack of concentration the problem is compounded, especially when a woman is unaware of why this is happening.

Both forgetfulness and loss of concentration are very common symptoms of perimenopause, also. In both conditions, hypothyroidism and perimenopause, the lack of ability to concentrate combined with a faulty memory make it difficult to organize one's thinking or establish priorities. Whether this fuzziness is due to a thyroid insufficiency or perimenopause, women often report feeling overwhelmed and incompetent as they find it a challenge to accomplish that which they easily accomplished in the past.

Frequently these cognitive impairments not only include difficulty focusing but bring on bothersome headaches. Together these symptoms may cause a woman to be concerned she has a brain tumor or some other severe neurological problem. Others may worry they have Alzheimer's Disease or dementia. How severe these symptoms become depends on how hypothyroid the individual is, how perimenopause is unfolding-or the combination of the two.

Another factor that affects the severity of cognitive symptoms is mood. High levels of anxiety or depression will worsen the cognitive deficits, whether they are due to the thyroid function or perimenopause. Struggling with cognitive impairment is a terribly upsetting situation for someone to experience, especially when the condition has not yet been appropriately diagnosed. Thankfully, treatment is simple. All that is needed to reverse hypothyroidism is a tiny daily pill or two of Thyroxin (T4) and/or Triiodothyronine (T3) to supplement one's thyroid hormone levels. This artificial thyroid hormone replacement will make all of the symptoms resulting from the thyroid problems disappear.

Emotional Symptoms

In the emotional realm, depression is an enormous challenge for the hypothyroid woman. There are too many stories of women who felt severely depressed, went to their doctors and were referred for psychotherapy without the doctor checking their thyroid hormone levels. *Statistics show that 15 percent of patients diagnosed with depression are hypothyroid.* An underactive thyroid wreaks havoc with moods and often leaves women feeling frightened and confused as to why they are feeling so down. Simple, everyday tasks can be overwhelming. The tendency for women suffering with an underactive thyroid is to put off or postpone their obligations to a day when they are "feeling better." Since this day never comes, the obligations begin to pile up. Ultimately they begin to feel very helpless which eventually leads to hopelessness. This is a potent trigger for depression. When hypothyroidism is treated, the depressed, sad, hopeless feelings from thyroid disease disappear. If there is a concomitant depression, the symptoms resulting from the depression will remain and will require alternative treatment.

Another symptom the hypothyroid woman has to manage is low libido. This is usually a function of the fatigue and lethargy caused by the underactive thyroid.[219] In fact, many of the symptoms are due to the slowing of the metabolism that is a result of the underactive thyroid, all of which resolve once the hypothyroidism is treated.

After having learned about both hypothyroidism and perimenopause, one can easily understand how many of these symptoms are shared between both conditions (see Table 26-1). A symptomatic woman in her forties or fifties may be suffering from one or both of these difficulties. It is apparent how confusing it can be to identify what truly is going on.

Thyroid Mary

Mary had a fine life. Her three children were grown, all attending or finished with college. She had a warm and loving marriage with the man she had fallen in love with as a young woman. She was very close with her parents and siblings, with whom she spent a lot of pleasurable time. Mary worked part time in a family run business and had plenty of time to enjoy the pleasures of tennis. She was active in community affairs. She kept herself fit and involved.

In her late forties Mary began to notice changes in her menstrual cycle. Her periods were heavier and less regular. Occasionally, she would skip a period. Mary knew that she was "starting her changes" and that this often brought with it some discomfort but Mary was feeling utterly miserable. Over the course of several months, Mary gained weight despite her tennis workouts and dieting. She always felt chilled, dressing more warmly than those around her. This confused her because all of her girlfriends were constantly having hot flashes. What was most difficult was her relentless fatigue. She no longer had the energy to keep pace with her life. Taking care of her home and family was a tremendous hardship. Everything was overwhelming. Mary became increasingly depressed.

Initially Mary's doctor felt this was all due to perimenopause. After several months of Mary feeling so poorly, her doctor decided to check her thyroid. The resulting blood work indicated Mary was hypothyroid. The treatment was simple. Mary was given replacement thyroid hormone, a daily pill, and within six months her thyroid levels were back to normal. Most of her symptoms lessened dramatically. The symptoms that remained were due to perimenopause, not a thyroid condition.

Mary continued to have her moods swings with her menstrual cycle. She still had to watch her diet to maintain her weight but she no longer had the relentless lethargy. Her body temperature normalized. In fact, she joined her girlfriends and began having hot flashes. Mary needed to be monitored for thyroid hormone levels as she progressed through perimenopause to menopause. Two years later, when Mary completed menopause, her thyroid hormone levels stabilized and Mary was comfortable on a regular dose of medication.

Table 26-1

Symptoms of Hypothyroidism and Perimenopause

	Hypothyroidism	Perimenopause
Metabolic		
Fatigue	X	X
Hypersensitivity to Cold	X	
Loss of Appetite	X	
Slow Heart Rate/Pulse	X	
Weight Gain	X	X
Heavy, Irregular Menstruation	X	X
Fertility Problems	X	X
Constipation	X	
Slowed Reflexes	X	
Susceptibility to Respiratory Infections	X	
Lowered Immune System	X	
High Cholesterol	X	X
Slowed Metabolism	X	X
Physical		
Hair Loss	X	X
Muscle Cramps	X	X
Numbness in Extremities	X	
Dry, Thinning Hair	X	X
Swollen Eyes	X	
Dry, Flaky Skin	X	X
Facial Puffiness	X	
Brittle, Peeling Fingernails	X	X
Husky Voice	X	

Migraines	X	X
Worsening of PMS Symptoms	X	X
Cognitive		
Difficulty Concentrating	X	X
Poor Memory	X	X
Decreased Intellectual Ability	X	X
Emotional/Psychological		
Depression	X	X
Fatigue	X	X
Low Libido	X	X
Feeling of Hopelessness	X	X
Feelings of being Overwhelmed	X	X
Inertia	X	X

Chapter Twenty-seven

Hyperthyroidism– Metabolic, Physical, Cognitive and Emotional Symptoms of an Overactive Thyroid

Women who are hyperthyroid (have an overactive thyroid) have an excess of thyroid hormone in their systems. This is the opposite of hypothyroidism in which there is insufficient thyroid hormone. One would intuit that all of the symptoms of hyperthyroidism would be the opposite of hypothyroidism but this is not always the case. This chapter will explain the differences and similarities of symptoms and the reasons for them, along with the symptoms of perimenopause that overlap with the symptoms of hyperthyroidism (Table 27-1).

Metabolic Changes

Women who have hyperthyroidism suffer an overabundance of thyroid hormone that results in a speeding up of their metabolisms. The excessive thyroid hormone increases the number of beta-adrenergic receptors, important in the functioning of adrenal hormones. These additional beta-adrenergic receptors raise the heart rate to create a rapid and forceful heartbeat. The heart rate may climb to 120[220] or even 150[221] beats per minute, up from the normal heart rate of 70 to 80 beats per minute.

This rapid heart rate may cause palpitations. Palpitations resulting from hyperthyroidism are different from the occasional, normal palpitations that can be present in euthyroid people. In those with normal thyroid function occasional palpitations may be experienced when they engage in physical exertion or stimulating substance use, such as caffeine. In hyperthyroid people the palpitations will present in relaxing situations such as sleeping or reading in addition to situations involving exertion.

The increase in beta-adrenergic receptors also causes hyperthyroid people to become much more sensitive to and thus more affected by their own adrenalin. The increase in this characteristic of adrenalin effect is implicated in many of the symptoms of hyperthyroidism.

The sped-up metabolism of hyperthyroidism has a number of other effects. Ramona, who was suffering from hyperthyroidism for nearly a year before being diagnosed, experienced a sense of impending danger and high anxiety as her metabolism raced. She was chronically prone to restlessness and insomnia. Even though hyperthyroidism involves a speeding up of the metabolism and body functions, a hyperthyroid individual will often feel exhausted because the body cannot keep pace with the increased level of activity. This was the case with Ramona. Her energy levels declined as a result of her overworked metabolism. Chronic insomnia and the resulting sleep deprivation contributed to her exhaustion. This physical energy drain plays a huge role in the psychological and emotional challenges of hyperthyroidism that will be discussed later in this chapter.

Opposite to the effects of hypothyroidism, hyperthyroid women will experience an increased speed of digestion with a change in bowel habits. Bowel movements will increase in frequency. There is commonly weight loss as the metabolism speeds up, regardless of whether the hyperthyroid individual is maintaining a highly caloric diet. The speeding metabolism also creates a fine tremor in the fingers or hands, an obvious symptom of too much thyroid hormone in the body. Logically, the severity of all of these symptoms is a function of how mild or extreme the hyperthyroidism is.

Because their bodies are running at an increased rate, hyperthyroid people will be very uncomfortable in warm environments, feeling hot or overheated most of the time. Their body temperature may actually be higher than 98.6 degrees. Ramona frequently felt her skin was damp and sweaty. In the forty to fifty year old woman this symptom is often mistaken to be a result of perimenopause because of the similarity to hot flashes.

Similar to hypothyroidism, hyperthyroidism adversely affects the menstrual cycle and may decrease fertility. *Opposite* to hypothyroidism, when a woman is hyperthyroid her periods become lighter and shorter. She may skip periods altogether. This, too, may be confused with the symptoms of perimenopause. You can refer back to Chapter 4 for a refresher on some of the menstrual cycle changes in perimenopause.

Menstrual irregularities, anxiety and insomnia are common to both hyperthyroidism and perimenopause in similar patterns and may cause confusion when trying separate the overlapping symptoms of these conditions. Diagnosis of hyperthyroidism is easy when one is looking for it. A simple blood test will yield accurate results that will allow for appropriate treatment.

Physical Symptoms

The physical effects of hyperthyroidism cause disruptions in many of the same areas as hypothyroidism but not always in opposite ways. Hair responds similarly to both hypothyroidism and hyperthyroidism by becoming finer and thinner. In an individual with hyperthyroidism, as in hypothyroidism, you may find clumps of hair falling out, or a general thinning on the scalp. Curly hair may straighten, dark hair become gray and hair may not respond to styling, coloring or perming as it normally would.

The way in which fingernails and toenails are affected by hyperthyroidism is by a speeding up of nail growth. When the nails grow faster, they are much softer and more easily torn. Fingertips may swell and occasionally the fingernails may begin to separate from the fingertips.

Some people may be familiar with the look of bulging eyeballs in severely hyperthyroid individuals. This is because the eyelids retract in the presence of significant and prolonged hyperthyroidism. The eyeball may protrude and the skin around the area of the eyes may swell giving the appearance of bulging eyes with a staring gaze.

A dangerous effect of excess thyroid hormone in the body is a wasting effect on the skeletal muscles leaving them weak and sore. It can also negatively impact bone density. This, in conjunction with the exhaustion and fatigue of the overworked metabolism in the hyperthyroid woman, can make simple activities difficult and painful. When Ramona learned of the risks of sustained hyperthyroidism, she was grateful she had seen her doctor and was diagnosed before any irreversible consequences evolved.

Once again we can see the overlap between symptoms of thyroid dysfunction and perimenopause. Hair loss, brittle fingernails, loss of bone density and general fatigue are common to both of these conditions.

Cognitive Symptoms

Hyperthyroidism in women does not appear to create cognitive changes as in the case of hypothyroidism. When the metabolism is sped up, the thought processes do not seem to be negatively affected.

Emotional Symptoms

While there are no notable cognitive changes, the emotional and psychological effects of hyperthyroidism can be quite profound. As the metabolic rate of the body speeds along, the individual experiences extreme exhaustion as physical and mental energy stores are drained. The body is incapable of providing the energy needed to keep up with the runaway metabolism. The speeding metabolism leaves the hyperthyroid woman feeling irritable, nervous, restless and edgy. Finding a time or a place where she can feel calm and relaxed will be an impossible undertaking because the pressure is metabolically driven and not a result of external issues.

Anxiety is a common feeling in hyperthyroid women, especially before the hyperthyroidism has been diagnosed. This was the symptom that initially brought Ramona to her doctor. She felt as though she was "coming out of her skin." This was atypical for Ramona who was generally a very calm and easy-going woman. The adrenergic system involved in hyperthyroidism, described at the beginning of this section, is the same system involved in Anxiety Disorders and panic disorders. The adrenalin is pumping, the body is in a state of alarm and the internal experience of the individual is that of danger and fear. When she is unaware that her metabolism is hormonally induced to race, the hyperthyroid woman may interpret this unusual feeling as quite frightening, resulting in anxiety and panic. Add to this the lack of sleep that is symptomatic of hyperthyroidism and the effect multiplies. Irritability and exhaustion continue to spiral out of control especially since even in sleep the metabolism continues to race, leaving the individual feeling exhausted upon awakening.

The effect of hyperthyroidism on a woman's libido is variable. Some women experience an increased sex drive because of the thyroid hormone's impact on the brain. Other women, because of the menstrual changes and overall exhaustion may experience a reduction in their sexual desires.[222] All of these effects are nerve-wracking and frightening. There appears to be no way for the hyperthyroid woman to achieve a feeling of wellbeing. Many women have reported feeling as if they are going crazy or worry they are losing their minds when in a hyperthyroid state.

Hyperthyroidism is a bit more difficult to treat than hypothyroidism. There are a number of treatments for hyperthyroidism including surgery to remove some part of the thyroid, beta-blockers, drugs that can reverse the effects of temporary hyperthyroidism, antithyroid drugs, or radioactive iodine. Today, the most common treatment option for long term or permanent hyperthyroidism is treatment with radioactive iodine. This is sometimes referred to as "medical thyroidectomy" because the thyroid gland is made partially inactive by the administration of a radioactive "cocktail" that is imbibed.[223] Once the hyperthyroidism has been diagnosed and treated, most effects disappear and the individual quickly returns to normal.

Table 27-1

Symptoms of Hyperthyroidism and Perimenopause

	Hyperthyroidism	Perimenopause
Metabolic		
Intolerance to Heat	√	√
Insomnia	√	√
Sleeplessness	√	√
Frequent Bowel Movements	√	
Speeding Up of Digestion	√	
Decrease in Flow, Frequency and Duration of Menses and Menstruation	√	√
Fatigue	√	√
Weight Loss	√	
Rapid Heartbeat/Increased Pulse Rate	√	
Palpitations	√	√
Infertility	√	√
Physical		
Excessive Perspiration	√	√
Weakness	√	√
Loss of Muscle Strength	√	√
Loss of Muscle Mass	√	√
Hair Loss	√	√
Hair becomes Finer	√	√
Weakened Nails	√	√
Speeding of Nail Growth	√	
Separation of Nails from Nailbed	√	
Tremors in Hand and Arms	√	
Protrusion of Eyeballs	√	

Decreased Bone Density	√	√
Increased Risk of Cardiovascular Disease	√	√
Joint Aches	√	√
Cognitive		
There are no obvious cognitive signs of hyperthyroidism		
Emotional/Psychological		
Nervousness	√	√
Irritability	√	√
Anxiety	√	√
Panic Attacks	√	√
Exhaustion	√	√
Shift in Libido	√	√
Restlessness	√	√
Depression	√	√
Agitation	√	√

Chapter Twenty-eight
Partners in Crime:
Estrogen and Thyroid Hormone

*B*ecause of the similarity of certain perimenopausal symptoms to those of hypothyroidism and hyperthyroidism, thyroid disease may be overlooked in the perimenopausal woman. This can put women at higher risks for other diseases, both physiological and psychological. The physiological complications are beyond the scope of *The Fifth Decade*; we will instead focus just on the psychological. It is apparent from the sections above, that the effects of unbalanced thyroid hormone have powerful influences on psychological health. Depressive Disorders, bipolar disorders, Anxiety Disorders and panic disorders can all be confused with the symptoms of thyroid disorders. To make matters more complex, some of the symptoms of these psychological disorders are frequently present in perimenopause. It is easy to recognize how complex the picture is for middle-aged women who are just not feeling right. It is a challenge to sort through the various hormonal and psychological impingements at this juncture in life.

Noreen's Tipping Point

Noreen had been a thyroid patient for many years. She was kept in a slightly hyperthyroid state through medication, as a treatment for a prior bout with thyroid cancer. This is a standard practice for people who have had a total thyroidectomy (removal of the thyroid gland) due to cancer. Noreen was accustomed to existing in this hyperthyroid state and was well versed on the side effects of hyperthyroidism. For this reason, she took, as needed, a low dose of a mild sleeping pill when she felt agitated and had trouble falling asleep.

At one point, with some surprise, Noreen realized that she had been taking the sleeping pill far more than usual; she had been using it nightly for several weeks. She rationalized that she had been under some additional stress recently but also realized that the "typical" stressors seemed to be affecting her more than usual. Nonetheless, Noreen decided she had better stop the sleeping medication before she became dependent on it.

What ensued became a very frightening event for Noreen. When she stopped taking the sleeping pill, she was unable to sleep. This not only concerned her tremendously but without sleep it was impossible to function in her very busy life. Noreen resigned herself to relying on the sleeping medication just a bit longer until her stress subsided. To her dismay, Noreen was no longer able to sleep without or with the medication. After several nights of sleeping 3 hours or less, Noreen wound up in the emergency room, in a highly anxious state, convinced she must have either a brain tumor or was losing her mind.

Noreen's CAT scan was unremarkable but the blood work drawn in the hospital did indicate that Noreen was severely hyperthyroid. Since Noreen had always prided herself on being well educated in matters of her own health and was diligent on following up on her appointments to assess her thyroid hormone levels, this news came as quite a shock. She had been on the same dosage *of thyroid hormone supplement for over ten years. Why was there a problem all of a sudden? What Noreen and the doctors were unaware of was that perimenopause was well underway. Her estrogen levels had dropped and this caused a complete unbalancing of her previously stable thyroid hormone levels.*

The fact that thyroid disease is fairly common in women who are also in perimenopause provides a difficult challenge. As noted earlier, during perimenopause, estrogen levels are fluctuating, often in a highly variable, unpredictable fashion. When estrogen levels are low, the female body requires less thyroid hormone. When estrogen levels are high, the body requires more thyroid hormone. In fact, when hypothyroid women become pregnant causing their estrogen levels to increase, they require on average, an increase of 45 percent or even 50 percent in their dose of thyroid replacement hormone.[224, 225, 226] Because of this interaction between estrogen and thyroid hormone, it is actually possible to use estrogen therapy in hyperthyroid women to moderate some of the effects of hyperthyroidism.[227]

This fluctuation in estrogen was the source of Noreen's problem. Her estrogen levels had dropped significantly as she progressed through perimenopause. This caused a reduced requirement for thyroid hormone. Because all of her thyroid hormone was supplied artificially, there was no mechanism for her body to respond accordingly as it would in women with a functioning thyroid. Unfortunately for Noreen, she was given a neurological exam and an exhaustive psychiatric evaluation before anyone thought to check her thyroid hormone levels. It was quite some time before her various medical doctors figured out the connection between her estrogen levels and her thyroid hormone levels. Once this was understood, Noreen's thyroid hormone supplements were adjusted. She was also put on a regimen of bioidentical hormone supplementation to help mitigate the fluctuations of perimenopausal hormones.

There are some complications when a perimenopausal woman is on replacement thyroid hormone. Replacement thyroid hormone is a wonderful fix for an underactive thyroid. However, replacement thyroid hormone is made to create a very steady blood level of thyroid hormone over the course of weeks. Even though it is taken daily, this medication will last in the blood stream for a long time. Again, in a normal, straight forward situation this is ideal. In a challenging situation, such as peri-menopause, the artificial supplementation of thyroid hormone cannot be responsive to the fluctuating need for thyroid hormone, leaving the woman temporarily hypo- or hyperthyroid at any given time.

In women with healthy, functioning thyroids, the thyroid responds to the changing demands in the body for thyroid hormone, regardless of the erratically changing needs due to the fluctuating estrogen levels. Within hours, days, weeks or months the estrogen levels will vary widely. The healthy thyroid will keep apace. The trouble starts when the thyroid is not healthy. Women who are hypothyroid will be unable to produce enough thyroid hormone when the body requires it.

The gap between what the body needs and can produce widens when the estrogen levels are high and the body needs even more thyroid hormone. At this juncture, a woman will be feeling quite hypothyroid, meaning she will be feeling pretty awful, with many of the symptoms described earlier. When her estrogen levels drop, her symptoms of hypo-thyroidism may ease a bit but she is then dealing with the effects of the lower estrogen. In one study, postmenopausal women with hypothyroid-ism that were being treated with estrogen, required additional thyroid hormone in order to maintain adequate thyroid hormone levels. The postmenopausal women in this study with normal thyroid function, who were also treated with estrogen, secreted the additional thyroid hormone from their thyroid glands.[228] It is apparent that estrogen and thyroid hor-mone require a delicate balance in order for a woman to feel her best.

When a woman is hyperthyroid and is in perimenopause she may have an experience similar to Noreen's. The severity of her symptoms will depend on how responsive her thyroid is. When her estrogen levels drop, she will need less thyroid hormone. If her thyroid is unhealthy, overproducing thyroid hormone, she will become even more hyperthyroid. She will feel the symptoms of hyperthyroidism described earlier; anxiousness, irritability, sleep difficulties and more. If her thyroid is at all responsive, her thyroid may be able to produce less thyroid hormone alleviating the severity of the hyperthyroid symptoms. The situation will be slightly better when her estrogen levels climb because the body will require more thyroid hormone; her thyroid levels become closer to what the body requires.

There has been some discussion over when in the menstrual cycle thyroid hormone levels should be measured. Thyroid hormone levels are screened by measuring the amount of TSH (thyroid stimulating hormone) in the blood. Current research indicates that TSH fluctuates least during days two to seven of the menstrual cycle. TSH concentrations have been reported to be higher during the luteal phase of the menstrual cycle, or the days from ovulation to menstruation.[229, 230] The higher the TSH concentration, the lower the levels of thyroid hormone in the body and vice versa; the lower the TSH values, the higher the levels of thyroid hormone in the body. Depending on when the blood tests are done, the determination of how to treat a potential problem may be variable. When there is a concern over the presence of abnormal thyroid function, especially in a perimenopausal woman, it is wise to take several measurements at different times in the menstrual cycle before implementing treatment.

Part IV

FOR THE MEN

This section offers a feature that many books on perimenopause and midlife changes do not; it speaks to the man's perspective on what is happening to the woman in his life. The goal is to give the husband or partner enough information to understand the challenges the woman is experiencing and how these changes affect him. To complete this section, I have interviewed many men from twenty-two to eighty-five years of age. Children, friends, coworkers and others in the lives of middle-aged, perimenopausal women frequently share the husbands' perspectives and experiences. For simplicity's sake, I will use the term "husband" to represent the many others that journey through this transition with women.

Chapter Twenty-nine

Who Are You and What Have You Done with My Wife?

Peter came in for his first session alone. He started off by asking, with a moan, how much longer it would take for his wife, Sherri, to be done with perimenopause. He just was not sure if he would be able to survive her "crazy" behavior much longer; the marriage was in jeopardy.

Peter was the sole breadwinner in the family. His job as a salesman was intense and demanding. He coped with his stress in a very passive way, primarily by not coping at all but by shoving everything inside. He prided himself on his even temperament and on not bringing home to his family the pressures of his job. The only outward sign of Peter's stress was occasional sarcasm or a sharp edge in his tone of voice. Peter dealt with the difficulties in life by disconnecting from the feelings they produced or from the person creating those feelings. When Sherri was in the throes of perimenopause, disconnection was no longer a viable option. It made a difficult situation unbearable because disconnection was the opposite of what Sherri needed.

Initially, Peter was perplexed about the changes Sherri was displaying. She did not react as he had come to expect after fifteen years of marriage. Typically, although a very emotional person, Sherri would react calmly and rationally when there were disagreements or discord between family members. She was very self-sufficient and confident as a homemaker, wife and mother. In the last few years, Peter began to observe an intensity and a high level of reactivity in Sherri that simply had not been there before. What was happening? Who was this person?

I had met Sherri about six months prior, when she had first come in alone. She talked about not feeling like herself. She was already somewhat familiar with the challenges of the perimenopause she was enduring, but primarily she was upset about the state of her marriage. Sherri acknowledged that she had less patience for her teenage children and found herself yelling a lot, but insisted that the problems in the marriage were primarily Peter's fault. She felt that he gave her little of what she needed and she was just not willing to live that way any longer. Peter and Sherri began fighting constantly. There was peace in the household only when Sherri and Peter kept their distance from one another. Their marriage was in serious trouble. Not only were they on the verge of divorce, their children were swept right into the chaos that was swirling throughout the whole family.

Most men have a limited knowledge of the difference between perimenopause and menopause, as if they are the same event. They may be aware that women have hot flashes and that their menstrual cycles stop. Some men are even aware that women may even be a little moody. Most men do not concern themselves with much beyond those simple bits of information. This is a mistake because the women in their lives may turn everything they have come to rely upon upside down and inside out.

What Men Need to Know About Perimenopause

Women in their late thirties to early forties begin to experience subtle shifts in the typical pattern of how their female hormones are released. The major players in perimenopausal changes are estrogen and progesterone. Typically, estrogen and progesterone work within a woman's body in shifting ways, but ways that balance each other. In perimenopause, this balance initially begins to wobble and eventually collapse, creating the emotional havoc so typical in perimenopause. (A detailed discussion of these hormonal changes can be found in Chapters 1 and 2.) The symptoms of perimenopause will worsen through the middle to late forties before beginning to abate, usually in the late forties to early fifties. The most important fact that men need to know is that the hormonal physiology will significantly affect the emotions, psychology and behavior of women.

Before perimenopause, estrogen is responsible for building the centers of the brain that involve communication, observation and nurturing. When estrogen is present in stable, moderate amounts, women have a healthy positive mood, adequate energy and normal libido. As perimenopause gets underway and estrogen begins to fluctuate wildly, is lowered or withdrawn, mood stability and libido deteriorate notably. If we think of female hormones in football terms, we can think of estrogen as the offense. Healthy estrogen levels make a healthy offense. A woman with appropriate, stable estrogen will be ready for a good game and proactive in setting up her "plays." She moves forward with confidence, clarity, healthy memory, stability of moods and nurturance, showing her best performance.

Progesterone is the defense. When estrogen begins to "get aggressive" or begins to vacillate, the female body secretes progesterone that will keep in check the effects of fluctuating estrogen. Progesterone is the calming, "feel good" hormone. While the vacillating or declining estrogen makes a woman's moods erratic, progesterone is the opposing force, quieting her and mitigating the stressful consequences of the estrogen. The progesterone works to prevent the effects of the estrogen from getting too far afield. The estrogen acts like the running back, charging down the field, dodging right and left, unpredictable in where it will go next. Without something to oppose it, it will run wild. The progesterone, like the linebacker, tries to slow down the estrogen running back. Finally, the defensive tackle takes down the running back; the body unleashes the progesterone full throttle to stop the runaway estrogen.

Now perimenopause hits. Imagine a football game with a good offensive (estrogen) team. In fact, this imaginary team has an extra four players on the field. This represents the excessive levels of estrogen present in the early stages of perimenopause. We have a great center snapping the ball back to the quarterback. The wide receiver catches the ball and the running back begins his run down the field. The extra players create a bit of chaos since their positions are confusing, generating more than usual activity on the field. This is similar to the chaos created by estrogen levels run amok. There is more than there ought to be and the consequences are confusing at a minimum and disastrous at worst. Emotionally, our perimenopausal woman does not know what to do, where to turn and how to cope when her estrogen levels are creating such havoc with her emotions. Her emotions are erratic- happy one moment, crying the next and ready to make heads roll a moment later.

The defense is in serious trouble since not only are there four extra players on the offense, but only two players show up for the defensive team. Let us remember that the defense represents progesterone. A woman in perimenopause produces less and less progesterone as perimenopause progresses, represented by having only two players on the defense. The defensive linebacker tries to stop the action but he barely creates an effect. The defensive tackle does not have a chance of catching the running back with only one other teammate on the field. The estrogen offensive is running wild. There is no way to stop it! The defense is helpless against the offense, just as progesterone can no longer protect a woman's emotional volatility against the onslaught of estrogen.

What those around this "defenseless" woman will experience will not be pretty. She will likely have notable mood swings. The monthly rhythm of her body for the past thirty plus years becomes unpredictable. She will be angry, impatient, snippy, depressed, and anxious. She may not be as nurturing as she was previously. She may feel lethargic, weepy and frequently overwhelmed. Her sex drive will plummet. She will suffer from insomnia. She may exist in stark contrast to the woman she was before. No longer is she the calm, comforting woman who led the family emotionally. She will now leave everyone around her feeling as lost and confused as she feels. No one, not even she can recognize her(self) anymore. Chapter 6 describes, in depth how the loss of progesterone affects women.

Men, like Peter, often feel rejected as their partners undergo such drastic changes. Peter complained that Sherri, his perimenopausal wife, would not care if he was alive or dead. This behavior is not because she has moved on, found another guy, fallen out of love or does not find him attractive anymore. It is because her hormones and her instincts are forcing her to turn inwards, to try to cope while going through this enormous change. It is also because she is emotionally stretched to the limit.

While in perimenopause, Sherri's most challenging and difficult behaviors always appeared to worsen in the two weeks prior to her starting her period. This is because perimenopause brings about a worsening of PMS. Even the educated, savvy, intuitive woman will be at the mercy of these challenges (See Chapter 4 for more information). One premenstrual woman, Eliza, was so irritated by her husband's frustrating question about where to find the barbeque sauce that she snapped at him with venom. When she saw the startled and hurt look on his face, *she* burst into tears. You can imagine how startled the look on his face was then!

Chapter Thirty

OK, I Will Take Directions,
Just Tell Me What To Do!

his is the time in their lives when men need to put aside their
pride and take directions. They have probably never felt more
lost than they do now. Many men have asked me a number of relevant
questions regarding how to handle their relationships with the perimenopausal women in their lives. I will share these questions and use them as
a guide for how to negotiate your way through this event.

How long does perimenopause last and when will it be over?

Perimenopause is the period of time that precedes menopause by up
to ten years. It begins very subtly, often when a woman is in her late thirties or early forties. By the time most women realize they are in perimenopause, they are more than half way through it. They will have completed
Stage I, Perimenopausal Initiation, and Stage II, Emotional Disruption.
(Read Chapter 10 for an understanding of the stages of perimenopause.)
The emotional symptoms are most severe in the third stage, Turbulence,
which is when you will notice most of the atypical (and often upsetting)

behaviors. Turbulence may last up to five years, but more typically it will last about three years. Turbulence finally gives way to Quietude, the end of perimenopause, which is much more peaceful. During Quietude, women are still menstruating irregularly, but the emotional rollercoaster has largely come to rest. Perimenopause is over when a woman has not had her period for one year.

How do I know if my partner is in perimenopause?

Some women are very open about changes happening in their bodies, some women are very private and others are in denial. If your partner is open, consider yourself fortunate. If your partner is private, you may have to work a bit harder to get the information. Forget about "TMI" (too much information) because every bit of information your perimenopausal partner gives you will be helpful in understanding what is going on and what she needs.

- When your partner tells you her period is changing, it is late, early or different in some way, this may be a sign of perimenopause. Every woman occasionally experiences some irregularities in her cycle, but when these differences become a regular event, you should take notice.
- When in perimenopause, a worsening of premenstrual symptoms (PMS) will occur in the week to two weeks before menses. This includes bloating, headaches, moodiness and/or fatigue. Women who have always had PMS will have it worse, while women who never had PMS may begin suffering from it.
- Perimenopause often brings insomnia. If your partner starts complaining of trouble falling asleep, frequent awakenings or awakening too early without falling back to sleep, she may be starting perimenopause.
- A reduction in enjoying nurturing may be another indication of changing hormones.

Jack's Confusion

One husband, Jack, was perplexed as he noticed that his forty-three year old stay-at-home wife, Elaine, no longer enjoyed fussing over the meals, home and children. This was a noticeable change since homemaking had always been Elaine's greatest pleasure. Jack was at a loss trying to understand how the woman he had known so well and for so long could suddenly seem like such a stranger.

- Mood swings and heightened emotionality is most likely *NOT* midlife onset of bipolar disorder. Look to the hormones!
- You wife may complain about: gaining weight, being unable to lose weight, thinning hair, having hot flashes or night sweats, sprouting some facial hair (do *NOT* offer her your razor) or simply not feeling like herself. You may notice she is more depressed or anxious than usual. These are all symptoms of perimenopause.
- Most women in their forties will be in some stage of perimenopause. There are women who begin early, in their thirties, and those who begin later in their forties. If the age is right and there are some of the changes mentioned above, chances are your lady is in perimenopause.

My wife denies being in perimenopause even though she has all of the symptoms. Maybe she is tired of me?

One forty-eight year old woman was sharing some of the "bizarre" changes happening in her body. When I suggested she might be in perimenopause, she looked at me in shock and exclaimed that there was no possible way; she was much too young! Some women have a very difficult time adjusting to the notion they may be entering this life-changing event. Keep in mind that menopause signifies the end of fertility. Some women feel that this diminishes their femininity and womanhood. Some have negative associations with other women, such as mothers and grandmothers who became "old" once they went through their "changes." These beliefs make it much more difficult to accept what is happening. If your wife is in denial, discretion and sensitivity will save you a lot of anguish.

Women in denial find it much easier to blame their struggles on someone else. It becomes more comfortable to attribute their bad moods to uncooperative children or a husband who does not help her enough. It is safer to blame a lowered sex drive on being overworked and under-appreciated. Frequently, perimenopausal women lash out at their spouses—blaming them for every frustration and unpleasant feeling. It is very difficult to accept that this is driven by an internal event. This does not mean it is your fault but she may be unable to see it any other way. Rather than insist her struggles are hormonally induced, try to be sympathetic to her complaints and give her time to accept what is happening. The irony is that if she believes the causes for her misery are from those around her, she has hope she can change her frustration by changing others. If her misery is internal, she has a difficult and frightening challenge with which to cope.

What are hot flashes and night sweats exactly?

It is not completely understood why perimenopausal women have hot flashes. It is believed that falling estrogen levels affect the thermoregulatory centers in the hypothalamus in the brain making it difficult for the body to regulate its temperature. In simple terms, changing estrogen levels make a woman's temperature regulation go haywire. To gain an understanding of what women experience, imagine this. It is a cold winter day and you are going to your buddy's house for a game of poker. You dress warmly, especially since your friend's house tends to be cold and drafty. You settle in at the poker table comfortably. Thirty minutes later it suddenly feels as if the temperature in the room is ninety degrees. You begin to sweat as the sensation of heat becomes intolerable. You cannot concentrate on the game because you are so extremely uncomfortable. You remove your sweater, looking around to see if anyone else is warm. No one seems to be having the same experience. As quickly as you felt hot, you now feel cold, even chilled. You grab your sweater to put it back on, because now the room feels like the sixty-five degrees it really is. Just as you settle back into your game, relieved that you feel comfortable, it starts all over again.

Hot flashes and night sweats can come in waves that are minutes apart, hours apart or days apart. Hot flashes are daytime "flushes" and night sweats are flushes that come during sleep. When they are frequent, women begin to become sleep deprived, irritable and sometimes anxious. You can see how hot flashes can make it so disruptive to living a peaceful and productive life.

What can I do to make it easier for her?

The formula for SUCCESS is as follows:

Support ... Be supportive. When she makes a request, try to accommodate her. Even simple tasks may seem overwhelming to her, so whatever you or the kids can do to ease her burden will be helpful and appreciated.

> *Mike survived his wife's mood swings by learning to use the washer/dryer. It helped her with her chores while he found an 'approved' way to escape!*

Understand ... Try to understand that she is going through something very foreign. She is as unhappy with her feelings and behavior as is everyone else. Keep in mind this is not something she has chosen.

Communicate ... Talk with her about what is happening. Ask her what is helpful and what is hurtful or difficult. Allow her to rail against the world if that is what she needs. Wait for the right moment to share your perspective with her.

Care ... Remind her that you care...even when you are completely at wit's end. You may have your rough moments but you love her enough to go the distance with her. Suggest she take some time for herself, whether it is to read a book, shop or just take a nap. This gives you the opportunity to grab a calm moment, too!

Empathy … Empathizing with female hormonal issues is no easy task for men because it is something they have never experienced. You may be able to gain a better understanding of what she feels like if you remember how you felt when you were coming down with the flu, while your boss was on your back, your favorite team lost the playoffs and your best friend broke your favorite, expensive tool—all at the same time—leaving you feeling sick, pressured, frightened, sad, frustrated and angry.

Snuggle … When all else fails, a nice snuggle works miracles. Taking some time out to hold her in your arms and let her feel that the world can be pushed aside for a few moments will be calming for her and an opportunity for connection with you.

Stroking … Non-sexual, tender stroking releases a hormone called oxytocin. Oxytocin is a very calming hormone that evokes relaxation and stress reduction by stimulating the pleasure centers in the brain (see Chapters 3 and 7). An offer of a massage when she is unduly challenged by her hormonal moods may be very much appreciated.

One husband, Brian found that whenever his wife, Bonnie, became stressed, a foot massage calmed her right down!

Keep in mind that for most women, perimenopause coincides with some other weighty life changes that burden the already overburdened. Some of these changes include children leaving the home, coping with the empty nest and redefining herself as someone other than "mom." Some women are also managing the needs of elderly parents with their requirements for additional help and support. The relationship between husband and wife will also experience strain as all of these moving parts create their effects.

It is so difficult to be around her. I would rather stay at work or go out with the guys.

Many men respond with avoidance when confronted with the emotional strains of female hormonal changes (See Chapter 7 for more information on the emotional strains associated with hormonal changes). It is perfectly logical that men will prefer to be in a world they find predictable and safe. Work, which offers a minimum of emotional entanglement and socializing, is often easy because men understand each other. The emotional range they share is much more limited and simpler than what they experience with women at home. While it is very important to have your "down time" with friends, be careful not to fall into a pattern of avoidance. That will only end up damaging your relationship by increasing feelings of isolation.

Joe began to ponder if his only option for happiness was with other men since he felt like a failure trying to relate to his adolescent daughter and perimenopausal wife—both on hormonal roller coasters!

My wife is never in the mood for sex anymore. Is this the end of our sex life?

Husbands of perimenopausal women are very upset by their wives' low libidos. Most women experience a huge drop in their sex drive as perimenopause gets under way. The direct effect of the changing hormones (lower estrogen and testosterone) along with the indirect effects (weight gain, exhaustion, poor body image, moodiness, etc.) can make a bid for sex feel like an unwelcome intrusion. (See Chapter 22 for more detailed information on changes to the libido.) While it is not a personal rejection, it is very hard for men not to experience it as one. Try to maintain physical intimacy in non-sexual ways when she is not in the mood for sex. Focus on sensuality over sexuality. She will be most receptive when she feels your hearts and minds are connected. Once she is past the worst of perimenopause, she will begin to regain her sexuality and will appreciate your patience while she was struggling.

What will she be like when this is over?

The majority of women emerge from perimenopause feeling better and happier with themselves than they have been in a long time. Some feel healthier and more confident than ever before. This means you will likely see an improved version of what you have always loved about her.

When she begins to feel settled and peaceful internally, she will also show that externally. This will be reflected in a return of—or even an increase in—her patience, tolerance and caring for her family and others. Quietude (see definition and explanation in Chapter 10), the final stage of perimenopause, brings women a sense of completeness and tranquility. They have survived a difficult journey ripe with changes that permeated every fiber of themselves, both physiologically and psychologically. Now they are ready to enjoy life again.

Chapter Thirty-one

Who is going to Take Care of Me?

Rather than panic or stress at the difficulties that lay in wait for them, husbands of midlife women can approach this time as one of learning, growth and empowerment for themselves. As you begin to comprehend the dynamics of perimenopause—including the reasons for your wife's outward withdrawal and aggression—you can stop blaming your wife *and* yourself. You can begin to differentiate selfishness from self-care or self-nurturance; something a woman desperately needs in order to help herself through this difficult time. This is the first step necessary for a man to begin taking care of himself. He is giving himself immunity from self-blame or feeling angry and miserable, now that he understands his wife is not treating him badly, but is displaying distress over what is happening within her.

Nonetheless, a man may still feel lost without the partner with whom he is accustomed to sharing his life. When a man approaches this transition in a healthy manner, it can provide an opportunity for substantial growth and development. He gets an opportunity to practice nurturing and patience as his wife did before perimenopause began. This can be a chance to learn how to tune in and sensitize himself to the nuances of his partner's mood. This does not imply that men have not been sensitive or nurturing previously, but this challenge presents the opportunity for a whole new level of empathic connectivity, something many men did not know they were capable of.

This personal growth gives men the confidence that not only can they take care of another, but that they can also fill the "care gap" now present in their relationship or within the family. When handled well, this can be a very empowering time for men. Men should keep in mind that as they begin to nurture their wives and learn how to take care of themselves, they will engender more emotionally reciprocal relationships. This will make her midlife transition easier for both, and for the rest of the family, as well.

Norm was in his mid-forties when his wife, Cindy, began to show the signs of perimenopause. He was completely unaware of this physiological event but was acutely aware that his wife was behaving very differently. Norm's distress became serious as he felt he could no longer please Cindy; everything he did brought criticism.

Norm and his wife started a family as older adults so they had school-age children when Cindy's changes took hold. When handling the children, the frustration Cindy sometimes experienced would bring her to tears or worse...hysterical crying jags. Norm witnessed Cindy's struggles and felt great concern, but whatever Norm tried to do to help seemed to make things worse. Eventually, it appeared the family was coming apart. The children became highly reactive to Cindy's erratic moods, yet she was less effectual in handling them. Norm was constantly on edge, feeling confused and helpless. He began spending more time at work, constantly looking for excuses to leave early and stay late. When he would come home, he would isolate himself by watching television or losing himself in his computer. It is no surprise that this resulted in a worsening of Cindy's attitude, as she felt abandoned and ignored.

Things began to turn around once Norm started to understand what Cindy was experiencing. To his credit, Norm began to understand that Cindy was not angry with him or unhappy with their life or children. She was undergoing a change that was as alien and uncomfortable to her as it was to everyone else, Norm, a bright and empathetic man became highly motivated to be supportive of his wife. Norm developed a strategy that included approaching Cindy in a caring manner rather than avoiding her when her moods seemed fragile or erratic. Cindy responded beautifully, as she learned she could lean on Norm when she felt off-kilter. As the family settled back into a more peaceful and functional rhythm, Norm experienced a sense of confidence and competence in the emotional interactions of his family that he had never experienced before. He became closer to his children and saw himself as a central figure in the family rather than the husband/father on the periphery.

As men gain comfort with this new-found emotional strength and competence, they may feel courageous enough to connect on a deeper level with their children. If the husbands have been feeling the strain from their wives' transition, so have their children. Stepping into that traditional "mom" role to engage and educate your children about mom's challenges will become another growth opportunity for men. This is no longer a "hush-hush" topic. Our culture is becoming much more comfortable talking openly about previously private matters. I am amazed at how many teenagers mention that they believe their mothers are "in menopause or something." Your wife and your children will appreciate having your participation when things get dicey between them, while you feel more confident with negotiating difficulties in an emotional realm.

Tom was very aware that his wife, Carol, was in perimeno-pause. Carol was knowledgeable about the changes happening to her and spoke openly with Tom about what she knew. Tom and Carol were coping fairly well with her changing emotions and perimenopausal difficulties until their daughter came home from college for the summer.

During the spring before and the summer her daughter was home, Carol was in the third stage of perimenopause—Turbu-lence. Turbulence is the most emotionally difficult stage for a woman. At times Carol felt close to being an emotional wreck, suffering from highly erratic mood swings. Tom and Carol's daughter, Chelsea, felt like she had come home to a "crazy house." Chelsea, having found a new sense of freedom and independence at college was ready for battle. She was intolerant of her mother's moodiness and was poised to fight with her over every request, expectation or obligation. With mom in Turbulence and Chelsea on the warpath, Tom was convinced it was, indeed, a crazy house!

As Carol and Chelsea's relationship deteriorated, along with every semblance of peace in the household, Tom knew he had to step in. Tom now became the voice of reason with Chelsea, where-as before Carol had always filled that role. Carol frequently saw Tom sitting on Chelsea's bed, speaking with her about her frustra-tions with mom. Tom was able to help Chelsea understand Carol's challenges, giving her the wisdom to increase her tolerance and empathy for her mother. Tom was happily amazed at how capable he was in dealing with these "female issues." He was filled with the pride of knowing that it was he who put the family back on the right path that summer.

When the situation gets too overwhelming, make sure to take some time for yourself. Exercising or having a social evening with friends or coworkers can offer a much needed break. Even the patience of the stron-gest of men will wear thin at times. I know men are not usually inclined to share feelings with one another, but discussing some of their experiences at this time may help them to normalize some of what is happening. Michael used humor in sharing with his buddies how he had to go to bed with long underwear, socks, a hat and sweatshirt because his wife's night sweats forced her to turn the thermostat down to sixty degrees! His friends and he wound up in a hilarious debate over whose wife froze which husband more!

Have patience, men. When the women in your life pass through this transition, they will resemble their former selves. The great majority of women feel even better about themselves after their changes than before this transition took hold. This translates into feeling more confident, tolerant and peaceful inside. When a woman, or anyone, for that matter, feels better about herself, those she loves will benefit from a far healthier and more positive relationship. When you and she know how hard you worked to learn, support and carry the family through a difficult time, you will feel the pride that you so deserve.

Words of Encouragement

The purpose of *The Fifth Decade* is to give people a clear understanding of the journey through the fifth decade of a woman's life. This knowledge is important for women, their husbands, children, friends and everyone with whom she shares a close relationship. While this journey may be trying at times, the challenges are made easier by having a greater understanding of what to expect, what is normal and how the changes progress.

It is commonplace for people to expect hot flashes and crankiness in the perimenopausal woman, but too few understand the emotional demands women suffer through and with which her loved ones have to cope. It is most helpful to understand this transition as a process. With the proper knowledge, understanding and interventions, the process becomes one through which women pass to attain a calm, integrated peace within themselves and with those they love. When things appear most hopeless, it is critical to remember that this is a natural transition in life through which all women must pass. Every emotion, every struggle and

every change associated with perimenopause and these years in the forties and fifties is fertilizer for positive growth into a happier and healthier
woman. In the end, women will rediscover themselves as being the same,
yet different.

The Author's Story

*It is four fifteen in the morning. I am lying in my daughter's bed
with my arm encircling her. In a soft, soothing voice, I am using
visual imagery to describe the comfortable, safe, protected feeling
she had when I carried her as an infant in the pouch on my chest.
She came home from college today, upset, needing to be home. She
awakened me a half hour ago crying, with acute insomnia. I grog-
gily got up and did what mothers do.*

*As my little baby twenty-year-old drifts off to sleep, I listen to
her breathing become deep and steady. I slowly get up to return
to my own bed when she whimpers, "mommy, stay." I recall the
many nights when she was an infant. I would get her settled down
into her crib and as soon as I began to tiptoe out of her bedroom,
she would begin to wail. Once again, twenty years later, I returned to hold her and comfort her until sleep took over.*

*Everything was the same, yet everything was different. As she
lay in my arms, I felt that familiar heat begin to rise up, first my
back, then my neck, until it engulfed all of me. Within moments,
it felt as if I was in a furnace. Ah, another night sweat. This trig-
gered my reflection on when so many difficulties began five years
before. When my daughter, my youngest, was in her junior year of
high school, I started down that slippery slope of worrying about
who I would be when the last of my children had left the nest.
I was in the throes of Turbulence (the third stage of perimenopause) feeling the emotional ups and downs, with the "downs"
being much more common. This was especially the case when I
dwelled upon the anticipated loss of my identity when my years of
"mothering" would be over. During her junior and senior years of*

high school, this fear continued to increase. My only comfort was to tell myself I had my very fulfilling career as a psychologist in which to immerse myself.

In my daughter's bed, in the wee hours of the morning, firmly entrenched in Quietitude, the final stage of perimenopause, and hopefully a mere few months away from menopause, I saw so clearly that I had really lost nothing, only gained. My child still needed me. I was still "mom," the same, yet different. I was here with her and for her but instead of worrying about dirty diapers, skinned knees or college applications, I was thinking about the coming deadline for this book. I had made the transition from the woman I was before to the woman I was now. I had journeyed through all of the stages of perimenopause. I had struggled with the life challenges that threatened my identity. I grew into someone new while retaining the someone old. I could now embrace myself completely as a woman—the moods, hot flashes, changes to my body and my thinking. My being a mother, therapist, wife, sister, daughter and friend was all a part of who I was, contributing to who I would be, complete with all of the emotions and all of the growth. I had survived the worst of my forties and was OK…even better than OK. I was content.

$\mathcal{A}ppendix$ *I*
Hormone Testing

$\mathcal{T}$he savvy woman of today who thinks she may be experiencing the first stirrings of perimenopause is likely to be exposed to all sorts of diagnostic tools to make this determination. A brief foray into a web search will offer her a multitude of home test kits recommending testing for any and all sex hormones. These kits include testing for estradiol, estrone and estriol, FSH, LH, progesterone DHEA and testosterone. Kits are offered at prices from $40 to over $200.

While hormone testing can be helpful, it has its limitations. Woman need to understand this in order to get a true sense of what is happening to them. Take the example of Shelly. Shelly had many of the "typical" symptoms of early perimenopause. She immediately ran out to buy a home test kit. This kit, which measured LH, a hormone that rises late in perimenopause, (unbeknownst to Shelly) claimed to determine if a woman is perimenopausal. When the results were negative, Shelly panicked that she was "losing it" because now her severe mood swings were unexplained.

Although on paper these changes seem very straightforward, in reality the hormonal shifts at this time in a woman's life can fluctuate widely and frequently. This can make it extremely difficult to get a handle on what is going on. The various methods of hormone testing are grossly inadequate in determining women's hormonal status. This is not because the blood and saliva tests that are available do not measure what they are supposed to measure. It is because a woman's hormonal levels can be vastly different within the course of days or even hours.

Blood testing for estrogen and progesterone levels is an inaccurate type of hormone testing because the majority of the hormone measured by the standard blood test is inactive. The active form of the hormones enters the body's tissues, and hence is not in the bloodstream, making the blood test inaccurate. Saliva hormone testing, on the other hand, more accurately reflects the hormone levels present in the body's tissues. Women who opt for saliva testing typically will give several samples at similar times of the day, over the course of several days, in order to reduce variability from her changing hormone cycles.

It is much easier to determine whether or not a woman has entered menopause than perimenopause. A simple blood test that measures FSH and or LH can be a good indicator of entry into late perimenopause or menopause. Testing the FSH may be indicated in a woman over the age of forty who is experiencing some of the common symptoms of perimenopause. Such symptoms may include menstrual irregularities, hot flashes, mood irregularities or other symptoms. These hormones are subject to fluctuation in perimenopause, thus requiring repeated testing to make that determination. If the perimenopause is in its early stages, the FSH levels may be normal and indicate nothing. *If* FSH testing is done, it should be conducted between the second and fifth days after the start of menstrual bleeding for the most accurate results. Even done this way, an FSH test may indicate perimenopause some months and not other months.[231]

A normal premenopausal level of these hormones may not indicate the absence of perimenopause, but an elevated level is very informative.

Both FSH and LH levels rise as menopause is underway, with FSH being the first to show elevated levels.[232] LH levels typically begin to rise later in the menopause transition. Eventually when a woman is one to three years postmenopausal, her LH levels will be three times what they were premenopausally and her FSH levels will peak at a ten- to twenty-fold increase.

A daily diary to track bodily changes is a comprehensive method to identify changes in your cycle and symptoms. You can make your own checklist of changes by referring to the many symptoms listed throughout *The Fifth Decade,* or you can use charts such as can be found at *www.cemcor.ubc.ca.*

Appendix II
Effects of Stress on the Adrenal Glands

*A*fter years of driving themselves at a frenetic pace, women begin to wear down. Emotionally they are drained. Physically, their adrenal glands become exhausted, creating an environment in the body in which it becomes hard to recover from the daily stresses. The adrenal glands function to produce three major hormones that are critical in the maintenance and homeostasis of stress and stress-related damage to the body.

Epinephrine

The first of these three hormones is epinephrine. People often talk about the "fight-or-flight" hormone. This is epinephrine, also called adrenaline. Epinephrine served humans very well when they were primitive people, living in the jungles and a tiger was bearing down on them. Epinephrine got the body moving. It gives the body a "rush"; it gets the heart pumping, blood rushing into various organs such as the heart, brain and lungs, and into the muscles. It sharpens the senses and gets a person ready to fight or flee from the danger. It makes us energized and focused.[233]

Historically, the instances of danger that released these huge surges of adrenaline were sporadic in nature. Today's "dangers" take a very different form. Epinephrine, or adrenaline is released throughout the day in response to the constant, stressful demands of modern day life. The traffic delays that make you late for work or for picking up the children from school or daycare will create an adrenaline surge. The deadline coming up for your project at work, the repairman showing up an hour late to fix your washing machine, the school nurse paging you while you are in a meeting because your child is sick, or your husband calling to say he has to travel for business next week, all induce the secretion of adrenaline. In today's hectic lifestyle, the adrenaline may be secreted on a continual basis as we experience one stressor after another. There is no battle to wage or tiger to run from to disperse the pent up energy, resulting in a calm aftermath. There is no endpoint to the danger. Living this way for a prolonged period of time will exhaust the adrenal glands.[234] They cannot keep up with this continual demand.[235]

Cortisol

The second of the adrenal hormones is cortisol. Cortisol is commonly referred to as the "stress hormone." When a woman is under constant, abundant stress, her adrenals begin to secrete an excess of cortisol. According to Brizendine,[236] cortisol's effect on a woman's brain is to make it "frizzled, frazzled, stressed out; highly sensitive, physically and emotionally."

The beneficial functions of cortisol are stimulating appetite, increasing energy and reducing inflammation. It aids the body in managing the stresses of trauma, infections and extreme temperatures. During pregnancy, high levels of cortisol in the brain increase the soon-to-be-mom's vigilance regarding her health, safety and nutrition in order to optimize the health of her unborn child.

So, when does cortisol become the frazzling hormone that Brizendine describes? When a woman is under continual, chronic stress her
adrenal glands are constantly secreting cortisol, a hormone meant to be
secreted only occasionally. When an excess of cortisol is released it will
create irritability and even fury. In women, cortisol has the effect of cutting off sexual desire. (In men, cortisol has the opposite effect, that of
increasing sexual desire.)

Cortisol is supposed to be a reserve system for energy, not the constant fix to a highly demanding lifestyle. The sort of relentless stress that
causes a chronic overproduction of cortisol results in adrenal exhaustion
and symptoms of chronic fatigue syndrome.[237] Eventually, the body will
no longer be able to maintain the production of cortisol at the level de-
manded for it.

Overproduction of cortisol also creates havoc in the body in indirect
ways. Because cortisol competes with progesterone for receptors in cells,
it actually interferes with the action of progesterone and creates an environment of estrogen dominance. Remember the symptoms of estrogen
dominance discussed in Chapter 8. Estrogen dominance creates havoc
in the woman's body in many ways from decreasing libido, to increasing
symptoms of PMS. It contributes to weight gain, mood swings, fatigue,
metabolism irregularities, headaches and also increases the risks of developing cysts and fibroids in the female organs. Estrogen dominance, as
a result of overproduction of cortisol, is also a main contributor to the
development of depression and anxiety. Lee and Hanley[238] describe this
cycle of how estrogen and stress combine to cause estrogen dominance.
The estrogen dominance, in turn, causes insomnia and anxiety. The insomnia and anxiety begin to exhaust the adrenal glands even further,
causing a worsening of the estrogen dominance.

Continuous high levels of cortisol also interfere with maintaining
healthy levels of blood sugar. The method by which cortisol gives the rush
of energy to the body is by sending glucose into the cells. This creates a
short-term period of vigor. As the blood sugar levels drop, you will feel
lethargic as you experience a drop in energy levels. You will crave more

and more sugar to re-invigorate yourself. Satisfying this urge is how cortisol becomes a factor in weight gain. Stress raises the cortisol levels in the body. The high cortisol levels send glucose flooding into the bloodstream. You feel a surge of energy and a burst of productivity. This is short-lived as the blood sugar levels fall off. The exhausted adrenals cannot keep pumping out the cortisol.

This is when the urge to forage for high sugar foods kicks in. You will eat what you can find in order to bring the blood sugar levels back up. If this is not troublesome enough, when the level of glucose in the blood is raised, the body is signaled to release more adrenaline, which in turn signals the production of more cortisol.[239]

This is how you wind up in a vicious cycle of *stress-cortisol production—blood sugar swings—production of more adrenaline*, with the resulting increase in stress and anxiety. Eventually, there is exhaustion, both physical and emotional.

Now that we understand the physiology of adrenaline and cortisol, we need to understand how this impacts us psychologically. In a fascinating study in which healthy young **men** were given estradiol (one of the estrogens), it was found that these men experienced increases in several stress hormones, including cortisol. Their stress response was stronger and lasted longer than in a control group.[240] This study illuminates the process of how each hormone or chemical in the body impacts another, changing the emotional experience of the individual.

DHEA

The third adrenal hormone that has a major involvement in stress related issues is referred to as DHEA, which is an abbreviation for dehydroepiandrosterone. DHEA is present in inverse proportion to cortisol in the body. When cortisol levels are high, DHEA levels are low, and vice versa. DHEA operates to help in the rebound of stressful impacts on the body, including extremes of temperature, pressures and illness. It actually improves the immune system by working in an antagonistic manner to cortisol.

DHEA is a steroid hormone, also produced in the adrenal glands, that helps maintain healthy sleep patterns, improves bone density, helps in maintaining cognitive acuity, a healthy libido and gives people energy and vigor. Not only does the production of DHEA become compromised as the adrenal glands become exhausted, but levels of DHEA decline sharply with increasing age.[241] After age twenty-five, women's levels of DHEA decline by approximately two percent each year. It is safe to assume that by the time a woman reaches her late forties her DHEA levels are very low,[242] and lower still when considering a woman who has been under the constant, relentless stress that results in the type of compromised adrenal function described above.

About the Author

$\mathscr{D}$eborah Wagner, Ph.D. earned her doctorate in Developmental Psychology from Yeshiva University. After receiving her doctorate she received the post-doctoral faculty appointment of Associate Research Scientist at Columbia University College of Physicians and Surgeons. While a post-doctoral scientist, Dr. Wagner researched the bonding, development and emotional wellbeing of women and their children. Her research was shared with the scientific community through professional publications and presentations at scientific conferences. Subsequently, she opened a successful clinical practice which has been thriving for over twenty years.

As both a researcher and a practicing psychologist, Dr. Wagner has been committed to achieving a greater understanding of how and why people feel and behave the way they do and has used these insights to help them find ways to feel and do better. She has dedicated her career to understanding the psychological ramifications of lifespan development and its impact on human emotions and reactions.

Dr. Wagner has worked in a clinical setting with individuals, couples and families from the ages of two through the eighties. From a clinical perspective, she has written on issues of parenting, child development and perimenopause and has created and currently authors the website *yourmentalhealth.info*.

Dr. Wagner currently lives in Northern New Jersey with her husband and a houseful of four-legged "children."

References

1   Minkin, M. (2006, June). Grand rounds: The art and science of managing perimenopause. *Contemporary OB/GYN. ModernMedicine.com*

2   Monroe, J.A., & Ledyard, R.H. (2001). Clinical Decision Making During the Perimenopause. *Hospital Physician*, 55-68.

3   Prior, J.C. (1998). Perimenopause: The complex endocrinology of the menopausal transition. *Endocrine Reviews*, 19(4), 397-428.

4   Prior, J.C. (2002). The ageing female reproductive axis II: ovulatory changes with perimenopause. In: Chadwick DJ, Goode JA, editors. Endocrine Facets of Ageing. 242 ed. Chichester, UK: John Wiley and Sons Ltd., 172-86.

5   Prior, J.C. (2002). The ageing female reproductive axis II: ovulatory changes with perimenopause. In: Chadwick DJ, Goode JA, editors. *Endocrine Facets of Ageing.* 242 ed. Chichester, UK: John Wiley and Sons Ltd., 172-86.

6   Prior, J.C. (1998). Perimenopause: The complex endocrinology of the menopausal transition. *Endocrine Reviews*, 19(4), 397-428.

7   Prior, J.C. (1998). Perimenopause: The complex endocrinology of the menopausal transition. *Endocrine Reviews*, 19(4), 397-428.

7   Cohen, L.S., Soares, C.N., & Joffe, H. (2005). Diagnosis and management of mood disorders during the menopausal transition. *The American Journal of Medicine*, 118, (12B), 93S-97S.

9   Prior, J.C. (1998). Perimenopause: The complex endocrinology of the menopausal transition. *Endocrine Reviews*, 19(4), 397-428.

10 Lee, J.R., & Hanley, J.R. (2009). *What Your Doctor May Not Tell You about Premenopause.* New York: Warner Books.

11 Prior, J.C. (1998). Perimenopause: The complex endocrinology of the menopausal transition. *Endocrine Reviews,* 19(4), 397-428.

12 Brizendine, Louann. (2006). *The Female Brain.* New York: Morgan Road Books.

13 Brizendine, Louann. (2006). *The Female Brain.* New York: Morgan Road Books.

14 Overlie, I., Moen, M.H., Morkrid, L., Skjaeraasen, J.S., & Holte, A. (1999). The endocrine transition around menopause-a five years prospective study with profiles of gonadotropines, estrogens, androgens and SHBG among healthy women. *Acta Obstetricia et Gynecologica Scandinavica,* 78, 642-647.

15 Gruber, C.J., Tshugguel, W., Schneeberger, C., & Huber, J.C. (2002). Production and actions of estrogens. *NEJM,* 346(5), 340-352.

16 Mason, J.W., Taylor, E.D., Brady, J.V. & Tolliver, A. (1968). Urinary estrone, estradiol, and estriol responses to 72-hr avoidance sessions in the monkey. *Psychosomatic Medicine,* XXX(5), 696-709.

17 Prior, J.C. (1998). Perimenopause: The complex endocrinology of the menopausal transition. *Endocrine Reviews,* 19(4), 397-428.

18 Cohen, L.S., Soares, C.N., & Joffe, H. (2005). Diagnosis and management of mood disorders during the menopausal transition. *The American Journal of Medicine,* 118, (12B), 93S-97S.

19

20 Freeman, E.W., Sammel, M. D., Lin, H., & Nelson, D.B. (2006). Associations of hormones and menopausal status with depressed mood in women with no history of depression. *Archives of General Psychiatry,* 63, 375-382.

21 Cohen, L.S., Soares, C.N., Poitras, J.R., Prouty, J., Alexander, A.B., & Shifren, J.L. (2003). Short-term use of estradiol for depression in perimenopausal and postmenopausal women: A preliminary report. *The American Journal of Psychiatry,* 160, 1519-1522.

22 Lee, J.R., & Hanley, J.R. (2009). *What Your Doctor May Not Tell You about Premenopause.* New York: Warner Books.

23 Mason, J.W., Taylor, E.D., Brady, J.V., & Tolliver, A. (1968). Urinary estrone, estradiol, and estriol responses to 72-hr avoidance sessions in the monkey. *Psychosomatic Medicine,* XXX(5), 696-709.

24 Brizendine, Louann. (2006). *The Female Brain.* New York: Morgan Road Books.

25   Brizendine, Louann. (2006). *The Female Brain*. New York: Morgan Road Books.

26   Brizendine, Louann. (2006). *The Female Brain*. New York: Morgan Road Books.

27   Meisler, M.S. (2003). Toward Optimal Health: The Experts Provide a Current Perspective on Perimenopause. *Journal of Women's Health*, 12(7), 609-615.

28   Prior, J.C. (1998). Perimenopause: The complex endocrinology of the menopausal transition. *Endocrine Reviews*, 19(4), 397-428.

29   Grady, Deborah. (2006). Management of Menopausal Symptoms. *NEJM*, 355(22), 2338-2347.

30   Hanisch, L., Hantsoo, L., Freeman, E., Sullivan, G., & Coyne, J. (2008). Hot flashes and panic attacks: A comparison of symptomatology, neurobiology, treatment, and a role for cognition. *Psychological Bulletin*, 134, (2), 247-269.

31   Meisler, M.S. (2003). Toward Optimal Health: The Experts Provide a Current Perspective on Perimenopause. *Journal of Women's Health*, 12(7), 609-615.

32   Thurston, R.C., Bromberger, J.T., Joffe, H., Avis, N.E., Hess, R., Crandall, C.J., Yuefang, C., Green, R., & Matthews, K.S. (2008). Beyond frequency: who is most bothered by vasomotor symptoms? *Menopause*, 15(5), 841-847.

33   Grady, Deborah. (2006). Management of menopausal symptoms. *NEJM*, 355(22), 2338-2347.

34   Moyer, P. (2004, May). Risk of depression increases during perimenopause. APA 157th Annual Meeting: Abstract NR768.

35   Kovacs, P. (2007, October). Conference Report. Highlights of the American Society of Reproductive Medicine 63rd Annual Meeting. Washington, DC.

36   Swartzman, L.C., Edelberg, R., & Kemmann, E. (1990). Impact of stress on objectively recorded menopausal hot flushes and on flush report bias. *Health Psychology*, 5, 529-545.

37   Monroe, J.A., & Ledyard, R.H. (2001). Clinical decision making during the perimenopause. *Hospital Physician*, 55-68.

38   Gruber, C.J., Tshugguel, W., Schneeberger, C., & Huber, J.C. (2002). Production and actions of estrogens. *NEJM*, 346(5), 340-352.

39   Hinson-Smith, V. (2002). Answering your questions about perimenopause. *Nursing*, 32(4), 14-16.

40   Hinson-Smith, V. (2002). Answering your questions about perimenopause. *Nursing*, 32(4), 14-16.

41   Prior, J.C. (1998). Perimenopause: The complex endocrinology of the menopausal transition. *Endocrine Reviews*, 19(4), 397-428.

42   Hinson-Smith, V. (2002). Answering your questions about perimenopause. *Nursing*, 32(4), 14-16.

43   Overlie, I., Moen, M.H., Morkrid, L., Skjaeraasen, J.S., & Holte, A. (1999). The endocrine transition around menopause-a five years prospective study with profiles of gonadotropins, estrogens, androgens and SHBG among healthy women. *Acta Obstetricia et Gynecologica Scandinavica*, 78, 642-647.

44   Brizendine, Louann. (2006). *The Female Brain*. New York: Morgan Road Books., Louann. (2006). *The Female Brain*. New York: Morgan Road Books.

45   Brizendine, Louann. (2006). *The Female Brain*. New York: Morgan Road Books.

46   Bromberger, J.T., Schott, L.L., Kravitz, H.M., Sowers, F., Avis, N.E., Gold, E.B., Randolph, J.F., & Mathews, K.A. Longitudinal change in reproductive hormones and depressive symptoms across the menopausal transition. (2010). *Archives of General Psychiatry*, 67, (6), 598-607.

47   Overlie, I., Moen, M.H., Morkrid, L., Skjaeraasen, J.S., & Holte, A. (1999). The endocrine transition around menopause-a five years prospective study with profiles of gonadotropins, estrogens, androgens and SHBG among healthy women. *Acta Obstetricia et Gynecologica Scandinavica*, 78, 642-647.

48   Brizendine, Louann. (2006). *The Female Brain*. New York: Morgan Road Books.

49   Prior, J.C. (2006). Perimenopause lost – reframing the end of menstruation *Journal of Reproductive and Infant Psychology*, 24(4), 323-335.

50   Gruber, C.J., Tshugguel, W., Schneeberger, C., & Huber, J.C. (2002). Production and actions of estrogens. *NEJM*, 346(5), 340-352.

51   Sherwin, B. Estrogen and cognitive functioning in women. (2003). Estrogen and cognitive functioning in women. *Endocrine Reviews*, 24(2), 133-151.

52   Brizendine, Louann. (2006). *The Female Brain*. New York: Morgan Road Books.

53   Brizendine, Louann. (2006). *The Female Brain*. New York: Morgan Road Books.

54   Thakur, M.K., & Sharma, P.K. (2006). Aging of brain: Role of estrogen. *Neurochemical Research*, 31, 1389-1398.

55   Gruber, C.J., Tshugguel, W., Schneeberger, C., & Huber, J.C. (2002). Production and actions of estrogens. *NEJM*, 346(5), 340-352.

56 Bromberger, J.T., Meyer, P.M., Kravitz, H.M., Sommer, B., Cordal, A., Rowell, L., Ganz, P.A., & Sutton-Tyrerell, K. (2001). Psychologic Distress and Natural Menopause. *American Journal of Public Health*, 91, 1435-1442.

57 Thakur, M.K. & Sharma, P.K. (2006). Aging of brain: Role of estrogen. *Neurochemical Research*, 31, 1389-1398.

58 Sherwin, B. Estrogen and cognitive functioning in women. (2003). Estrogen and cognitive functioning in women. *Endocrine Reviews*, 24 (2): 133-151.

59 Sherwin, B. Estrogen and cognitive functioning in women. (2003). Estrogen and cognitive functioning in women. *Endocrine Reviews*, 24 (2): 133-151.

60 Thakur, M.K., & Sharma, P.K. (2006). Aging of brain: Role of estrogen. *Neurochemical Research*, 31, 1389-1398.

61 Sherwin, B. Estrogen and cognitive functioning in women. (2003). Estrogen and cognitive functioning in women. *Endocrine Reviews* 24 (2): 133-151.

62 Sherwin, B. Estrogen and cognitive functioning in women. (2003). Estrogen and cognitive functioning in women. *Endocrine Reviews* 24 (2): 133-151.

63 Rapposelli, D. (2006). Distractions of life at crux of perimenopausal memory complaints. *Neurology*, 61, 801-806

64 Ohayon, M. (2006). Severe hot flashes are associated with chronic insomnia. *Archives of International Medicine*, 166 (12), 1262-1268.

65 Hinson-Smith, V. (2002). Answering your questions about perimenopause. *Nursing*, 32(4), 14-16.

66 Rosenthal, M. S. (2005). *The Thyroid Sourcebook for Women*. New York: McGraw Hill, 2005.

67 Mayo Clinic. Perimenopause. (2006). Perimenopause. *Mayoclinic.com/ health/perimenopause.*

68 Lee, J.R., & Hanley, J.R. (2009). *What Your Doctor May Not Tell You about Premenopause*. New York: Warner Books.

69 Wright, J.V., & Morganthaler, J. (1997). *Natural Hormone Replacement*. California: Smart Publications, 1997.

70 Lee, J.R., & Hanley, J.R. (2009). *What Your Doctor May Not Tell You about Premenopause*. New York: Warner Books.

70 Wright, J.V., & Morganthaler, J. (1997). *Natural Hormone Replacement*. California: Smart Publications, 1997.

71   Polo-Kantola, P., Saaresranta, T., & Polo, O. (2001). Aetiology and treatment of sleep disturbances during perimenopause and postmenopause. *CNS Drugs,* 15(6), 445-452.

72   Ohayon, M. (2006). Severe hot flashes are associated with chronic insomnia. *Archives of International Medicine,* 166(12), 1262-1268.

73   Maas, James B. (2001). *Power Sleep.* New York: Quill, M. Evans and Company, Inc.

74   Harvey, J. R. (2001). *Deep Sleep.* New York: M. Evans and Company, Inc.

75   Harvey, J. R. (2001). *Deep Sleep.* New York: M. Evans and Company, Inc.

76   Krystal, A.D. (2001). Insomnia in peri-menopausal and post-menopausal women. *Geriatric Times,* II (3).

77   Miller, E. (2005). Hormonal Changes and Insomnia in Perimenopause and Postmenopause. *Topics in Adult Primary Care—Insomnia Expert Column. Medscape Family Medicine,*7(1).

78   Kovacs, P. (2007, October). Conference Report. Highlights of the American Society of Reproductive Medicine 63rd Annual Meeting. Washington, DC.

79   Polo-Kantola, P., Saaresranta, T., & Polo, O. (2001). Aetiology and treatment of sleep disturbances during perimenopause and postmenopause. *CNS Drugs,* 15(6), 445-452.

80   Ohayon, M. (2006). Severe hot flashes are associated with chronic insomnia. *Archives of International Medicine,* 166(12), 1262-1268.

81   Polo-Kantola, P., Saaresranta, T., & Polo, O. (2001). Aetiology and treatment of sleep disturbances during perimenopause and postmenopause. *CNS Drugs,* 15(6), 445-452.

82   Thurston, R.C., Blumenthal, J.A., Babyak, M.A., & Sherwood, A. (2006). Association between hot flashes, sleep complaints, and psychological functioning among healthy menopausal women. *International Journal of Behavioral Medicine,* 13(2), 163-172.

83   Prior, J.C. (1998). Perimenopause: The complex endocrinology of the menopausal transition. *Endocrine Reviews,* 19(4), 397-428.

84   Thurston, R.C., Blumenthal, J.A., Babyak, M.A., & Sherwood, A. (2006). Association between hot flashes, sleep complaints, and psychological functioning among healthy menopausal women. *International Journal of Behavioral Medicine,* 13(2), 163-172.

85   Harvey, J. R. (2001). *Deep Sleep.* New York: M. Evans and Company, Inc.

86   Maas, James B. (2001). *Power Sleep.* New York: Quill, M. Evans and Company, Inc.

87   Maas, James B. (2001). *Power Sleep.* New York: Quill, M. Evans and Company, Inc.

88   Thurston, R.C., Blumenthal, J.A., Babyak, M.A., & Sherwood, A. (2006). Association between hot flashes, sleep complaints, and psychological functioning among healthy menopausal women. *International Journal of Behavioral Medicine*, 13(2), 163-172.

89   Polo-Kantola, P., Saaresranta, T., & Polo, O. (2001). Aetiology and treatment of sleep disturbances during perimenopause and postmenopause. *CNS Drugs*, 15(6), 445-452.

90   Harvey, J. R. (2001). *Deep Sleep*. New York: M. Evans and Company, Inc.

91   Harvey, J. R. (2001). *Deep Sleep*. New York: M. Evans and Company, Inc.

92   Krahn, L.E. (2005). Perimenopausal depression? Ask how she's sleeping. *Current Psychiatry*.com

93   Maas, James B. (2001). *Power Sleep*. New York: Quill, M. Evans and Company, Inc.

94   Prior, J.C. (2006). Perimenopause lost—reframing the end of menstruation *Journal of Reproductive and Infant Psychology*, 24(4), 323-335.

95   Freud, S. (1959). *Collected Papers* (Vol II) (p.-308). New York: Basic Books.

96   Freud, S. (1959). *Collected Papers* (Vol IV) (p.-139). New York: Basic Books.

97   Polo-Kantola, P., Saaresranta, T., & Polo, O. (2001). Aetiology and treatment of sleep disturbances during perimenopause and postmenopause. *CNS Drugs*, 15(6), 445-452.

98   Smith, A.(1998). The estrogen dilemma. *American Journal of Nursing*, 98(4), 17-20.

99   Brizendine, Louann. (2006). *The Female Brain*. New York: Morgan Road Books.

100   American Psychiatric Association. (1994). *Diagnostic and Statistical Manual of Mental Disorders*, Fourth Edition. Washington, DC, American Psychiatric Association.

101   American Psychiatric Association. (1994). *Diagnostic and Statistical Manual of Mental Disorders*, Fourth Edition. Washington, DC, American Psychiatric Association.

102   American Psychiatric Association. (1994). *Diagnostic and Statistical Manual of Mental Disorders*, Fourth Edition. Washington, DC, American Psychiatric Association.

103   American Psychiatric Association. (1994). *Diagnostic and Statistical Manual of Mental Disorders*, Fourth Edition. Washington, DC, American Psychiatric Association.

104   American Psychiatric Association. (1994). *Diagnostic and Statistical Manual of Mental Disorders*, Fourth Edition. Washington, DC, American Psychiatric Association.

105   Freeman, E.W., Guthrie, K.A., Caan B., Sternfeld, B., Cohen, L.S., Joffe, Carpenter, J.S., Anderson, G.L., Larson, J.C., Ensrud, K. E., Reed, S.D., Newton, K.M., Sherman, S., Sammel, M.D., & LaCroix, A.Z. (2011). Efficacy of escitalopram for hot flashes in healthy menopausal women. A randomized controlled trial. *JAMA,* 305 (3), 267-274.

106   DeAngelis, T. (2008) Psychopharmacology: When do meds make the difference? *Monitor on Psychology,* 39 (2).

107   Mazure, C. M., Keita, G.P., & Blehar, M.C. (2002, October). Summit on Women and Depression. American Psychological Association. Wye River Conference Center.

108   Moneysmith, M. Progesterone cream primer. (2007). *Better Nutrition,* 69(2), 24-27.

109   Ernst, Edzard. (2009). Herbal remedies for depression and anxiety. *Advances in Psychiatric Treatment,* 13 (4), 312-319.

110   Dennerstein, L., Guthrie J.R., Clark, M., Lehert, P., & Henderson, V. ((2004). A population-based study of depressed mood in middle-aged, Australian-born women. *The North American Menopause Society,* 11(5), 563-568.

111   Mazure, C. M., Keita, G.P., & Blehar, M.C. (2002, October). Summit on Women and Depression. American Psychological Association. Wye River Conference Center.

112   American Psychiatric Association. (1994). *Diagnostic and Statistical Manual of Mental Disorders*, Fourth Edition. Washington, DC, American Psychiatric Association.

113   American Psychiatric Association. (1994). *Diagnostic and Statistical Manual of Mental Disorders*, Fourth Edition. Washington, DC, American Psychiatric Association.

114   Mazure, C. M., Keita, G.P. & Blehar, M.C. (2002, October). Summit on Women and Depression. American Psychological Association. Wye River Conference Center.

115   American Psychiatric Association. (1994). *Diagnostic and Statistical Manual of Mental Disorders*, Fourth Edition. Washington, DC, American Psychiatric Association.

116   American Psychiatric Association. (1994). *Diagnostic and Statistical Manual of Mental Disorders*, Fourth Edition. Washington, DC, American Psychiatric Association.

117 American Psychiatric Association. (1994). *Diagnostic and Statistical Manual of Mental Disorders*, Fourth Edition. Washington, DC, American Psychiatric Association.

118 American Psychiatric Association. (1994). *Diagnostic and Statistical Manual of Mental Disorders*, Fourth Edition. Washington, DC, American Psychiatric Association.

119 Morgan, M.A., & Schulkin, J. (2006). Obstetrician-gynecologists and self-identified depression: personal and clinical. *Depression and Anxiety*, 23, 83-89.

120 Mazure, C. M., Keita, G.P., & Blehar, M.C. (2002, October). Summit on Women and Depression. American Psychological Association. Wye River Conference Center.

121 Aloysi, A., Van Dyk, K., & Sano M. (2006). Women's cognitive and affective health and neuropsychiatry. *The Mount Sinai Journal of Medicine*, 73(7), 967-975.

122 Mazure, C. M., Keita, G.P., & Blehar, M.C. (2002, October). Summit on Women and Depression. American Psychological Association. Wye River Conference Center., Keita & Blehar

123 Pearlstein, T.B. (1995). Hormones and depression: What are the facts about premenstrual syndrome, menopause, and hormone replacement therapy? *American Journal Obstetrical Gynecology*, 173(2), 646-653.

124 Cohen, L.S., Soares, C.N., & Joffe, H. (2005). Diagnosis and management of mood disorders during the menopausal transition. *The American Journal of Medicine*, 118, (12B), 93S-97S.

125 Freeman, E.W., Sammel, M.D., Liu, L., Gracia, C.R., Nelson, D.B., & Hollander, L. (2004). Hormones and menopausal status as predictors of depression in women in transition to menopause. *Archives of General Psychiatry*, 61, 62-70.

126 Morgan, M.A., & Schulkin, J. (2006). Obstetrician-gynecologists and self-identified depression: personal and clinical. *Depression and Anxiety*, 23,83-89.

127 Cohen, L.S., Soares, C.N., Vitonis, A.F., Otto, M.W., & Harlow, B.L. (2006). Risk for new onset of depression during the menopausal transition. *Archives of General Psychiatry*, 63(4), 385-390.

128 Cohen, L.S., Soares, C.N., & Joffe, H. (2005). Diagnosis and management of mood disorders during the menopausal transition. *The American Journal of Medicine*, 118,(12B), 93S-97S.

129 Sherwin, B. Estrogen and cognitive functioning in women. (2003). Estrogen and cognitive functioning in women. *Endocrine Reviews* 24(2): 133-151.

130 Pearlstein, T.B. (1995). Hormones and depression: What are the facts about premenstrual syndrome, menopause, and hormone replacement therapy? American *Journal Obstetrical Gynecology,* 173(2), 646-653.

131 Moyer, P. (2004, May). Risk of Depression Increases during Perimenopause. APA 157th Annual Meeting: Abstract NR768.

132 Harvard Women's Health Watch. (2006, November). Perimenopause, hormones, and midlife health. www.health.harvard.edu

133 Cohen, L.S., Soares, C.N., Vitonis, A.F., Otto, M.W., & Harlow, B.L. (2006). Risk for new onset of depression during the menopausal transition. *Archives of General Psychiatry,* 63(4), 385-390.

134 Deecher, D., Andree, T. H., Sloan, D., & Schechter, L.E. (2008). From menarche to menopause: Exploring the underlying biology of depression in women experiencing hormonal changes. *Psychoneuroendocrinology,* 33 (1), 3-17.

135 Cohen, L.S., Soares, C.N., & Joffe, H. (2005). Diagnosis and management of mood disorders during the menopausal transition. *The American Journal of Medicine,* 118, (12B), 93S-97S.

136 Pearlstein, T.B. (1995). Hormones and depression: What are the facts about premenstrual syndrome, menopause, and hormone replacement therapy? *American Journal Obstetrical Gynecology,* 173(2), 646-653.

137 Ozturk, O., Eraslan, D., Mete, H.E., & Ozsener, S. (2006). The risk factors and symptomatology of perimenopausal depression. *Maturitas,* 55(2), 180-186.

138 Cohen, L.S., Soares, C.N., & Joffe, H. (2005). Diagnosis and management of mood disorders during the menopausal transition. *The American Journal of Medicine,* 118, (12B), 93S-97S.

139 Cohen, L.S., Soares, C.N., & Joffe, H. (2005). Diagnosis and management of mood disorders during the menopausal transition. *The American Journal of Medicine,* 118, (12B), 93S-97S.

140 Cohen, L.S., Soares, C.N., Vitonis, A.F., Otto, M.W., & Harlow, B.L. (2006). Risk for new onset of depression during the menopausal transition. *Archives of General Psychiatry,* 63(4), 385-390.

141 Moyer, P. (2004, May). Risk of Depression Increases during Perimenopause. APA 157th Annual Meeting: Abstract NR768.

142 Pearlstein, T.B. (1995). Hormones and depression: What are the facts about premenstrual syndrome, menopause, and hormone replacement therapy? *American Journal Obstetrical Gynecology,* 173(2), 646-653.

143 Cohen, L.S., Soares, C.N., & Joffe, H. (2005). Diagnosis and management of mood disorders during the menopausal transition. *The American Journal of Medicine,* 118, (12B), 93S-97S.

144 Pearlstein, T.B. (1995). Hormones and depression: What are the facts about premenstrual syndrome, menopause, and hormone replacement therapy? *American Journal Obstetrical Gynecology,* 173(2), 646-653.

145 Mazure, C. M., Keita, G.P., & Blehar, M.C. (2002, October). Summit on Women and Depression. American Psychological Association. Wye River Conference Center.

146 Cohen, L.S., Soares, C.N., & Joffe, H. (2005). Diagnosis and management of mood disorders during the menopausal transition. *The American Journal of Medicine,* 118, (12B), 93S-97S.

147 Mazure, C. M., Keita, G.P., & Blehar, M.C. (2002, October). Summit on Women and Depression. American Psychological Association. Wye River Conference Center.

148 Harvard Women's Health Watch. (2006, November). Perimenopause, hormones, and midlife health. www.health.harvard.edu

149 DeAngelis, T. (2008) Psychopharmacology: When do meds make the difference? *Monitor on Psychology,* 39 (2).

150 Mazure, C. M., Keita, G.P., & Blehar, M.C. (2002, October). Summit on Women and Depression. American Psychological Association. Wye River Conference Center.

151 Monroe, J.A., & Ledyard, R.H. (2001). Clinical Decision Making During the Perimenopause. *Hospital Physician,* 55-68.

152 Gramann, S.B., & Lundquist, R.S. (2011). Menopause and mood disorders. *Emedicine.medscape.com.*

153 Lochner, C., Hemmings, S.M.J., Kinnear, C.J., Moolman-Smook, J.C., Corfield, V.A., Knowles, J.A., Niehaus, D.J.H., & Stein, D.J. (2004). Corrigendum to "gender in obsessive-compulsive disorder: clinical and genetic findings". *European Neuropsychopharmacology,* 14, 105-113.

154 Pacchierotti, C., Castrogiovanni, A., Cavicchioli, C., Luisi, S., Morgante, G., De Leo, V., Petraglia, F. & Castrogiovanni, P. (2004). Panic disorder in menopause: a case control study. *Maturitas,* 48, 147-154.

155 Smoller, J.W., Pollack, M.H., Wassertheil-Smoller, S., Barton, B., Hendrix, S.L., Jackson, R.D., Dicken, T., Oberman, A., & Sheps, D.S. (2003). Prevalence and correlates of panic attacks in postmenopausal women. *Archives of Internal Medicine,* 163, 435-445.

156 Gramann, S.B., & Lundquist, R.S. (2011). Menopause and mood disorders. *Emedicine.medscape.com.*

157 Basson, R. (2006). Sexual desire and arousal disorders in women. *NEJM,* 354 (14), 1497-1506.

158 Brizendine, Louann. (2006). *The Female Brain.* New York: Morgan Road Books.

159   Reed, S.D., Newton, K.M., Lacroix, A.Z., Grothaus, L.C., & Ehrlich, K. (2007). Night sweats, sleep disturbance, and depression associated with diminished libido in late menopausal transition and early postmenopause: baseline data from the Herbal Alternatives for Menopause Trial (HALT). *American Journal of Obstetrics & Gynecology,* 196 (6) 593-597.

160   Brizendine, Louann. (2006). *The Female Brain.* New York: Morgan Road Books.

161   Hinson-Smith, V. (2002). Answering your questions about perimenopause. *Nursing,* 32 (4), 14-16.

162   Monroe, J.A., & Ledyard, R.H. (2001). Clinical Decision Making During the Perimenopause. *Hospital Physician,* 55-68.

163   Reed, S.D., Newton, K.M., Lacroix, A.Z., Grothaus, L.C., & Ehrlich, K. (2007). Night sweats, sleep disturbance, and depression associated with diminished libido in late menopausal transition and early postmenopause: baseline data from the Herbal Alternatives for Menopause Trial (HALT). *American Journal of Obstetrics & Gynecology,* 196 (6) 593-597.

164   Basson, R. (2006). Sexual desire and arousal disorders in women. *NEJM,* 354 (14), 1497-1506.

165   Reed, S.D., Newton, K.M., Lacroix, A.Z., Grothaus, L.C., & Ehrlich, K. (2007). Night sweats, sleep disturbance, and depression associated with diminished libido in late menopausal transition and early postmenopause: baseline data from the Herbal Alternatives for Menopause Trial (HALT). *American Journal of Obstetrics & Gynecology,* 196 (6) 593-597.

166   Reed, S.D., Newton, K.M., Lacroix, A.Z., Grothaus, L.C., & Ehrlich, K. (2007). Night sweats, sleep disturbance, and depression associated with diminished libido in late menopausal transition and early postmenopause: baseline data from the Herbal Alternatives for Menopause Trial (HALT). *American Journal of Obstetrics & Gynecology,* 196 (6) 593-597.

167   Basson, R. (2006). Sexual desire and arousal disorders in women. *NEJM,* 354 (14), 1497-1506.

168   Monroe, J.A., & Ledyard, R.H. (2001). Clinical Decision Making During the Perimenopause. *Hospital Physician,* 55-68.

169   Sherwin, B. Estrogen and cognitive functioning in women. (2003). Estrogen and cognitive functioning in women. *Endocrine Reviews,* 24 (2) 133-151.

170   De Franciscis, P., Cobellis, L., Fornaro, F., Sepe, E., Torella, M., & Colacurci, N. (2007). Low-dose hormone therapy in the perimenopause. *Journal of Gynecology and Obstetrics,* 98, 138-142.

171   Inan, I., Kelekci, S., & Yilmaz, B. (2005). Psychological effects of tibolone and sequential estrogen-progestrogen therapy in perimenopausal women. *Gynecological Endocrinology,* 20 (2), 64-68.

172   Brizendine, Louann. (2008) Minding menopause: Psychotropics vs. estrogen? What you need to know now. *Current Psychiatry,* 2(10), 12-31.

173   Cohen, L.S., Soares, C.N., Poitras, J.R., Prouty, J., Alexander, A.B., & Shifren, J.L. (2003). Short-term use of estradiol for depression in perimenopausal and postmenopausal women: A preliminary report. *The American Journal of Psychiatry,* 160, 1519-1522.

174   Gruber, C.J., Tshugguel, W., Schneeberger, C., & Huber, J.C. (2002). Production and actions of estrogens. *NEJM,* 346_(5), 340-352.

175   Cicinelli, E. (2007). Bioidentical estradiol gel for hormone therapy in menopause. Expert Review of *Obstetrics & Gynecology,* 2(4), 423-430.

176   Lee, J.R., & Hanley, J.R. (2009). *What Your Doctor May Not Tell You about Premenopause.* New York: Warner Books.

177   Prior 2007

178   Moneysmith, M. Progesterone cream primer. (2007). *Better Nutrition,* 69(2), 24-27.

179   Wright, J.V., & Morganthaler, J. (1997). *Natural Hormone Replacement.* California: Smart Publications, 1997.

180   Freeman, E.W., Guthrie, K.A., Caan B., Sternfeld, B., Cohen, L.S., Joffe, Carpenter, J.S.,Anderson, G.L., Larson, J.C., Ensrud, K. E., Reed, S.D., Newton, K.M., Sherman, S., Sammel, M.D., & LaCroix, A.Z. (2011). Efficacy of escitalopram for hot flashes in healthy menopausal women. A randomized controlled trial. *JAMA,* 305 (3), 267-274.

181   Freeman, M. P., Hill, R., & Brumbach, B. H. (2006) Escitalopram for Perimenopausal Depression: An Open-Label Pilot Study. *Journal of Women's Health,* 15 (7), 857-861.

182   Kovacs, P. (2007, October). Conference Report. Highlights of the American Society of Reproductive Medicine 63rd Annual Meeting. Washington, DC.

183   Nelson, H.D., Vesco, K.K., Haney, E., Fu, R., Nedrow, A., Miller, J., Nicolaidis, C., Walker, M., & Humphrey, L. (2006). Nonhormonal therapies for menopausal hot flashes. Systematic review and meta-analysis. *JAMA,* 295(17), 2057-2071.,

184   Rovner, S.L. (2009). Hot flashes: Still a Mystery. *Science & Technology,* 87(47), 33-35.

185   Joffe, H., Petrillo, L., Viguera, A., Koukopoulos, A., Silver-Heilman, K., Rarrell, A., Yu, G., Silver, M. & Cohen, L.S. (2010). Eszopiclone improves insomnia and depressive and anxious symptoms in perimenopausal, and postmenopausal women with hot flashes: a randomized, double-blinded, placebo-controlled crossover trial. *American Journal of Obstetrics & Gynecology,* 202 , 171.e1-11.

186 Glazier, M.G., & Bowman, M.A. (2001), A review of the evidence for the use of phytoestrogens as a replacement for traditional estrogen replacement therapy. *Archives of Internal Medicine.* 161 (9), 1161-1172.

187 Nedrow, A., Miller, J., Walker, M., Nygren, P., Huffman, L.H., & Nelson, H. (2006). Complementary and alternative therapies for the management of menopause-related symptoms. *Archives of Internal Medicine,* 166 (14), 1453-1465.

188 Rotem, C., & Kaplan, B. (2007). Phyto-Female Complex for the relief of hot flushes, night sweats and quality of sleep: Randomized, controlled, double-blind pilot study. *Gynecological Endocrinology,* 23 (2), 117-122.

189 Nelson, H.D., Vesco, K.K., Haney, E., Fu, R., Nedrow, A., Miller, J., Nicolaidis, C., Walker, M., & Humphrey, L. (2006). Nonhormonal therapies for menopausal hot flashes. Systematic review and meta-analysis. *JAMA,* 295(17), 2057-2071.

190 Glazier, M.G., & Bowman, M.A. (2001). A review of the evidence for the use of phytoestrogens as a replacement for traditional estrogen replacement therapy. *Archives of Internal Medicine.* 161(9), 1161-1172.

191 Lie, D. (2006). AAFP-2006-Evidence-based complementary and alternative medicine (CAM): What should physicians know? American Academy of Family Physicians 2006 Scientific Assembly.

192 Hudson, T. (2002). Perimenopause and menopause alternatives to conventional HRT for symptom management-Women's Health Update. *Townsend Letter for Doctors and Patients.*

193 Nedrow, A., Miller, J., Walker, M., Nygren, P., Huffman, L.H., & Nelson, H. (2006). Complementary and alternative therapies for the management of menopause-related symptoms. *Archives of Internal Medicine,* 166 (14), 1453-1465.

194 Rachev, E., Nalbansky, B., Lolarov, G., & Agrosi, M. (2001). Efficacy and safety of phospholipid liposomes in the treatment of neuropsychological disorders associated with the menopause: a double-blind randomized, placebo-controlled study. *Current Medical Research and Opinion,* 17(2).

195 Bellipanni, G., Bianchi, P., Pierpaoli, W., Bulian, D. & Ilyia, E. (2001). Effects of melatonin in perimenopausal and menopausal women: a randomized and placebo controlled study. *Experimental Gerontology,* 36, 297-310.

196 Borud, E.K., Alraek, T., White, A., Fonnebo, V., Eggen, A.E., Hammar, M., Astrand, L.L., Theodorsson, E., & Grimsgaard, S. (2009). The acupuncture on hot flushes among menopausal women (ACUFLASH) study, a randomized controlled trial. *Menopause: The Journal of The North American Menopause Society,* 16(3), 484-493.

197   Kim, K.H., Kang, K.W., Kim, D., Kim, H.J., Yoon, H.M., Lee, J.M., Jeong, J.C., Lee, M.S., Jung, H.J., & Choi, S. (2010). Effects of acupuncture on hot flashes in perimenopausal and postmenopausal women-a multicenter randomized clinical trial. *Menopause: The Journal of The North American Menopause Society*, 17(2), 269-280.

198   Rowland, B., & Odle, T.G. (2005). Menopause. *Gale Encyclopedia of Alternative Medicine* 2, 1330-1335.

199   Nedrow, A., Miller, J., Walker, M., Nygren, P., Huffman, L.H., & Nelson, H. (2006). Complementary and alternative therapies for the management of menopause-related symptoms. *Archives of Internal Medicine*, 166 (14), 1453-1465.

200   Cohen, B.E. (2008). Yoga: an evidence-based prescription for menopausal symptoms? *Menopause*, 15(5), 827-829.

201   Chattha, R., Raghuram, N., Venkatram, P., & Hongasandra, N. (2008). Treating the climacteric symptoms in Indian women with an integrated approach to yoga therapy: a randomized control study. *Menopause: The Journal of The North American Menopause Society*, 15(5), 862-870.

202   Manocha, R., Semmar, B., & Black, D. (2007). A pilot study of a mental silence form of meditation for women in perimenopause. *Journal of Clinical Psychology in Medical Settings*, 14, 266-273.

203   Rowland, B., & Odle, T.G. (2005). Menopause. *Gale Encyclopedia of Alternative Medicine* 2, 1330-1335.

204   Chattha, R., Raghuram, N., Venkatram, P., & Hongasandra, N. (2008). Treating the climacteric symptoms in Indian women with an integrated approach to yoga therapy: a randomized control study. *Menopause: The Journal of The North American Menopause Society*, 15(5), 862-870.

205   Hanisch, L., Hantsoo, L., Freeman, E., Sullivan, G., & Coyne, J. (2008). Hot flashes and panic attacks: A comparison of symptomatology, neurobiology, treatment, and a role for cognition. *Psychological Bulletin*, 134, (2), 247-269.

206   Gramann, S.B., & Lundquist, R.S. (2011). Menopause and mood disorders. *Emedicine.medscape.com.*

207   Greendale, G.A., Huang, M., Wight, R.G., Seeman, T., Luetters, C., Avis, N.E., Johnston, J., & Karlamangla, A.S. (2009). Effects of the menopause transition and hormone use on cognitive performance in midlife women. *Neurology*, 72, 1850-1857.

208   Sowers, M.F., Luborsky, J., Perdue, C., Arajo, L.L.B., Goldman M.B., & Harlow, S.D. (2003). Thyroid stimulating hormone (TSH) concentrations and menopausal status in women at the mid-life: SWAN. *Clinical Endocrinology*, 58, 340-347.

209   Sowers, M.F., Luborsky, J., Perdue, C., Arajo, L.L.B., Goldman M.B., & Harlow, S.D. (2003). Thyroid stimulating hormone (TSH) concentrations and menopausal status in women at the mid-life: SWAN. *Clinical Endocrinology*, 58, 340-347.

210   Ain, K., & Rosenthal, M. S. (2005). *The Complete Thyroid Book*. New York: McGraw Hill.

211   Rosenthal, M. S. (2005). *The Thyroid Sourcebook for Women*. New York: McGraw Hill, 2005.

212   Ain, K., & Rosenthal, M. S. (2005). *The Complete Thyroid Book*. New York: McGraw Hill.

213   Hamburger, J.I., & Kaplan, M.M. (1997). *The Thyroid Gland: A Book for Thyroid Patients*, 7th ed. West Bloomfield, MI.

214   Sowers, M.F., Luborsky, J., Perdue, C., Arajo, L.L.B., Goldman M.B., & Harlow, S.D. (2003). Thyroid stimulating hormone (TSH) concentrations and menopausal status in women at the mid-life: SWAN. *Clinical Endocrinology*, 58, 340-347.

215   Sowers, M.F., Luborsky, J., Perdue, C., Arajo, L.L.B., Goldman M.B., & Harlow, S.D. (2003). Thyroid stimulating hormone (TSH) concentrations and menopausal status in women at the mid-life: SWAN. *Clinical Endocrinology*, 58, 340-347.

216   Rosenthal, M. S. (2005). *The Thyroid Sourcebook for Women*. New York: McGraw Hill, 2005.

217   Ain, K., & Rosenthal, M. S. (2005). *The Complete Thyroid Book*. New York: McGraw Hill.

218   Hamburger, J.I., & Kaplan, M.M. (1997). *The Thyroid Gland: A Book for Thyroid Patients*, 7th ed. West Bloomfield, MI.

219   Rosenthal, M. S. (2005). *The Thyroid Sourcebook for Women*. New York: McGraw Hill, 2005.

220   Hamburger, J.I. & Kaplan, M.M. (1997). *The Thyroid Gland: A Book for Thyroid Patients*, 7th ed. West Bloomfield, MI.

221   Ain, K., & Rosenthal, M. S. (2005). *The Complete Thyroid Book*. New York: McGraw Hill.

222   Ain, K., & Rosenthal, M. S. (2005). *The Complete Thyroid Book*. New York: McGraw Hill.

223   Hamburger, J.I., & Kaplan, M.M. (1997). *The Thyroid Gland: A Book for Thyroid Patients*, 7th ed. West Bloomfield, MI.

224   Surks, M.I., Sievert, R. (1995). Drugs and thyroid function. *NEJM*, 333(25), 1688-1694.

225   Arafah, B. M. (2001). Increased need for thyroxine in women with hypothyroidism during estrogen therapy. *NEJM*, 23, 1743-1749.

226 Toft, A. (2004). Increased levothyroxine requirements in pregnancy-why, when and how much? *NEJM*, 351(3), 292-294.

227 Arafah, B. M. (2001). Increased need for thyroxine in women with hypothyroidism during estrogen therapy. *NEJM*, 23, 1743-1749.

228 Arafah, B. M. (2001). Increased need for thyroxine in women with hypothyroidism during estrogen therapy. *NEJM*, 23, 1743-1749.

229 Sowers, M.F., Luborsky, J., Perdue, C., Arajo, L.L.B., Goldman M.B., & Harlow, S.D. (2003). Thyroid stimulating hormone (TSH) concentrations and menopausal status in women at the mid-life: SWAN. *Clinical Endocrinology*, 58, 340-347.

230 Overlie, I., Moen, M.H., Morkrid, L., Skjaeraasen, J.S., & Holte, A. (1999). The endocrine transition around menopause-a five years prospective study with profiles of gonadotropines, estrogens, androgens and SHBG among healthy women. *Acta Obstetricia et Gynecologica Scandinavica*, 78, 642-647.

231 Monroe, J.A., & Ledyard, R.H. (2001). Clinical decision making during the perimenopause. *Hospital Physician*, 55-68.

232 Prior, J.C. (1998). Perimenopause: The complex endocrinology of the menopausal transition. *Endocrine Reviews*, 19(4), 397-428.

233 Lee, J.R., & Hanley, J.R. (2009). *What Your Doctor May Not Tell You about Premenopause*. New York: Warner Books.

234 Ain, K., & Rosenthal, M. S. (2005). *The Complete Thyroid Book*. New York: McGraw Hill.

235 Brizendine, Louann. (2006). *The Female Brain*. New York: Morgan Road Books.

236 Brizendine, Louann. (2006). *The Female Brain*. New York: Morgan Road Books.

237 Lee, J.R., & Hanley, J.R. (2009). *What Your Doctor May Not Tell You about Premenopause*. New York: Warner Books.

238 Lee, J.R., & Hanley, J.R. (2009). *What Your Doctor May Not Tell You about Premenopause*. New York: Warner Books.

239 Lee, J.R., & Hanley, J.R. (2009). *What Your Doctor May Not Tell You about Premenopause*. New York: Warner Books.

240 Kirschbaum, C., Schommer, N., Federenko, I., Gaab, J., Neumann, O., Oellers, M., Rohdeder, N., Untiedt, A., Hanker, J., Pirke, K., & Hellhammer, D. (1996). Short-term estradiol treatment enhances pituitary-adrenal axis and sympathetic responses to psychosocial stress in healthy young men. *Journal of Clinical Endocrinology and Metabolism*, 81(10), 3639-3643.

241 Overlie, I., Moen, M.H., Morkrid, L., Skjaeraasen, J.S., & Holte, A. (1999). The endocrine transition around menopause-a five years prospective study with profiles of gonadotropines, estrogens, androgens and SHBG among healthy women. *Acta Obstetricia et Gynecologica Scandinavica, 78,* 642-647.

242 Lee, J.R., & Hanley, J.R. (2009). *What Your Doctor May Not Tell You about Premenopause.* New York: Warner Books.

Index

CPSIA information can be obtained at www.ICGtesting.com
Printed in the USA
LVOW061749091012

302146LV00012B/13/P